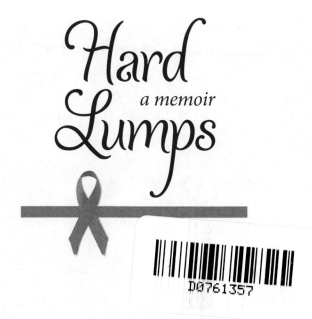

Hard
a memoir
Lumps

MIROLAND IMPRINT 3

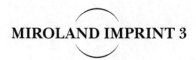

 Canada Council   Conseil des Arts
for the Arts   du Canada

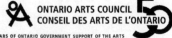
ONTARIO ARTS COUNCIL
CONSEIL DES ARTS DE L'ONTARIO
50 YEARS OF ONTARIO GOVERNMENT SUPPORT OF THE ARTS
50 ANS DE SOUTIEN DU GOUVERNEMENT DE L'ONTARIO AUX ARTS

Guernica Editions Inc. acknowledges the support
of the Canada Council for the Arts
and the Ontario Arts Council.
The Ontario Arts Council is an agency
of the Government of Ontario.

We acknowledge the financial support
of the Government of Canada through
the Canada Book Fund (CBF) for our publishing activities.

Hard Lumps

a memoir

Nancy-Gail Burns

MiroLand
p u b l i s h e r s

MIROLAND (GUERNICA)
TORONTO • BUFFALO • LANCASTER (U.K.)
2014

Michael Mirolla, general editor
Connie McParland, series editor
David Moratto, interior book design
Guernica Editions Inc.
P.O. Box 76080 Abbey Market, Oakville (ON) Canada L6M 3H5
2250 Military Road, Tonawanda, N.Y. 14150-6000 U.S.A.

Distributors:
University of Toronto Press Distribution,
5201 Dufferin Street, Toronto (ON), Canada M3H 5T8
Gazelle Book Services, White Cross Mills, High Town, Lancaster LA1 4XS U.K.

First edition.
Printed in Canada.

Legal Deposit — First Quarter
Library of Congress Catalog Card Number: 2013958127

Library and Archives Canada Cataloguing in Publication

Burns, Nancy-Gail, author
Hard lumps : a memoir / Nancy-Gail Burns.

(MiroLand ; no. 3)
Issued in print and electronic formats.
ISBN 978-1-55071-924-6 (pbk.).--ISBN 978-1-55071-925-3 (epub).--
ISBN 978-1-55071-926-0 (mobi)

1. Burns, Nancy-Gail--Health. 2. Breast--Cancer--Patients--
Canada--Biography. 3. Breast--Cancer--Patients--Canada--
Anecdotes. I. Title.

RC280.B8B87 2014   362.196'994490092   C2014-900025-1   C2014-900026-X

To my mother, Leona Burns, who taught me the meaning of working hard, and my father, Edward Burns, who magnified the magic within dreams.

S ATURDAY MORNING GROCERY shopping is for idiots, masochists, and bona fide cheapskates. Cars circle like sharks, as they hunt for a parking spot. A grey Mazda darts in front of me, seizing a spot designated for pregnant women. A tall, young man leaps from the vehicle. I suspect he is not pregnant. A blue Honda backs out. I pull in, as soon as I can clear its tail. I grab my bags, clench my teeth, and enter the store. People zoom by, snatching items off shelves. The gatherers, the hunters, are en force, even in the modern world. I am the ultimate bargain hunter. I fill my larder with reduced items. A stern looking woman jostles me as she reaches for peaches. I shove my cart in front of her, blocking her path. Butting in line is a faux pas. Pushiness does not deserve rewards.

Superstores are the rage. Aisles span for miles. I make my way down the gangway, as my eyes dart left and right. Countless grocery carts hit my heel, making it as fleshy as the rainbow trout that lured me in. People check their Blackberries, or are on their phones, or listen to music, or perhaps do all three. It's too taxing to notice the individuals around them. I observe the ... advancements. Saturday is not the day to venture out, because everyone has their head up their apps.

The rainbow trout baits me into coming because I'm a fish-eating cheapskate. I can't resist the weekend sale price. I save a monumental seven dollars. It's half price, but how much fish can one eat? As you can guess, I'm not a happy shopper. Hearing my name, okay not my name, but a nickname, I turn around and glare.

"Where are you off to in such a hurry, you little shithead?" the voice repeats.

I look up, way up, into the face of Darcy O'Grady. She's at least six foot one and built like a linebacker, but insists that she's five ten, and not even near the two hundred pound range. Right, and I have a body like a Barbie doll. Actually, I do, if you purchase the Asian model. You must have seen her. Flat chested and short. I'm getting off track. I'm also not Asian. Just flat chested and short. Let's talk about Darcy. She looks healthy, which is a compliment if you were once ill. Her auburn hair is mid length and shiny, her face round and pretty. Thick lashes frame her blue eyes. Arched brows look at me inquisitively. Darcy has a strapping body, a razor sharp mind, and a penchant for ultra feminine clothing. Today she's wearing a baby blue blouse, with ruffles dripping down to form a soft cascading collar. Her right hand clutches a dainty purse. It's vintage bark cloth in a blue floral pattern. Somehow, she carries off this dichotomy. Instead of complimenting, I quip: "By the looks of you, I assume the neighbourhood children still fear for their lives."

"I'll have you know I'm on a diet, and it's only the neighbourhood dogs and cats that have anything to worry about."

Before I can think of an insulting comeback, my head is wedged between two enormous breasts. I wheeze through a small crevice: "Let go of me, before my ribs crack."

Luckily, she obliges before I pass out.

Fellow shoppers stop and gawk at our encounter. The air is at *at-wention* (readiness for direct communication on twitter). When they realize a murder is not about to take place in aisle five, they retract their phones. No *twama*, (drama on twitter) nothing *intwesting* to fire off, so they carry on with their business. Is it just me, or has technology created a world of broadcasters, rather than doers? Is the human race taking a giant step backwards? Does it sound as if everyone speaks with a lisp?

Darcy scrutinizes me, before saying: "You're not looking as bad as usual."

I have lost weight, resurrected my exercise regime, and cut my hair absurdly short. I take no credit for that fashion statement. In a moment of maniacal inspiration, my hairdresser decides my small features are better suited with a short do. Hair flies to the floor like a troop of kamikaze pilots. I can only stare in abject horror. When the butchery is complete, a self-satisfied smile appears on her face. "You look ten years younger."

If you're over thirty-five, and they reduce your hair to stubble, they always employ the age ruse. The bigger the blunder, the younger you look. A decade constitutes a major gaffe. If she had bothered to ask, I would have told her: short hair is not an option, small features or not. Every morning after the haircut, I become the warden of an archaic insane asylum, forced to deal with an unrestrained uprising that demands hosing down the inmates, until they submit to normalcy. I pull at my hair, and hope the tugging will encourage it to grow.

"I feel good," I reply.

"I'm finished shopping. Once you're done, we can grab a cup of coffee next door. It'll be like old times."

Next door is a pretentious coffee shop that insists you order a cafe grande, instead of a large coffee. If you don't use their jargon, they pretend not to know what you want. They supposedly can't comprehend the unconventional lingo of small, medium, and large. I like to jerk them around, and refuse to imitate their terminology. They look at me as if I'm dim-witted. Repeated failed efforts to get me to say grande conclude with an exasperated sigh and a large coffee in my hand. To make matters worse, the coffee shop is crowded and overpriced. I hate that sort of place, but I return Darcy's smile, agree to meet her there, and hurry to the check out.

The lines are winding. The patrons sour faced, and surly. I head off to the self-serve.

"Take the last item out of the bag," the machine advises me. I have yet to remove an item from the cart.

Darcy is leaving the store. She waves and says: "I'll get us a table."

To understand my relationship with Darcy, and the other women I was lucky to enough to meet, I must start at the beginning. My words and thoughts may blur because I want to be truthful, and our history is awash with tears. Some are born out of sorrow, others of anger, some are happy, or relieved, and the remainder are of sheer frustration. For each of us found a hard lump and it forever changed our lives.

1

*D*OCTORS ARE NOT my favourite people. They tell you what you don't want to hear, and make you wait hours to hear it. Considering my lousy attitude, it's not surprising that my annual check-up only occurs when my doctor insists she will not refill my Lipitor, unless I book an appointment for a complete physical. It's a practise I call prescription blackmail, and it's highly effective. Heart attack versus seeing the doctor: Fine, I'll make an appointment.

After the common tests, Doctor Fungus (not her real name) remarks that she's going to check my breasts for lumps, bumps and things that make you yell ouch, when squeezed. I mention how I sometimes feel a pea sized bump in my right breast, but it's gone by the time I begin my menstruation.

"Probably a little cyst," she says, not having felt anything unusual. Nonetheless, when my exam is over, I hold a requisition form for a mammogram. "You're at that age," she explains as she bestows an extra bonus. I examine the kit to collect stool samples and stop myself from yelling yuk.

I take the requisition form and agree it's time to have my first mammogram. I smile as I assure her that I grasp the mechanics behind the stick and accompanying cardboard envelope, with its daily slots. It is an Advent calendar for grownups! Getting older opens doors I would prefer stayed closed.

Fifty is the new forty. Nonetheless, it still whispers you're not young anymore and things can go wrong. I don't mind being fifty, except when I shop for a bathing suit, or they ask me to bag my crap.

I leave her office, get into my car, and throw the forms into my purse. Once home, I throw them on my desk and forget about them for six weeks. In a moment of compliance, I decide Doctor Fungus is right. I call the clinic to book an appointment for the mammogram. I'm lucky; a cancellation allows me to come in the following day.

Small breasted, I've heard stories about how the test hurts like hell, especially when your playing field is level. Psychologically I prepare for it. It'll be over with quickly. I can then say I'm a good patient who does what is asked of her. Well, almost everything. I promise myself I'll start collecting stool samples on Monday. Monday is always my start day, especially with diets. Luckily, I have a poor memory and tend to forget about the task until at least Wednesday. I then wait to begin the following Monday. Do you see where this is going? But really, you have to refrigerate it.

"Mom where are the eggs?"

"Next to the advent calendar."

"No!!! Don't open the slots."

Time flies when you dread doing something. I find myself sitting in the clinic's vapid waiting room. The walls, the carpet, the chairs: all a mind-numbing beige. I suspect its tediousness is purposely designed to elicit listlessness. Compliance goes hand in hand with boredom.

"Nancy-Gail Burns," the receptionist calls out. She repeats herself, and gives everyone the stare down. On her third try, it dawns on me. I'm Nancy-Gail Burns. Stupefied, I follow the tall willowy blonde-haired woman into a room which holds a contraption that'll tell me if my breasts are normal.

The technician is a compact grey haired woman whose movements are sure and precise.

"Do you get tired of examining boobs all day?" I say.

Her face remains deadpan, as she says, chortling: "Could be worse. I could be examining assholes."

I enjoy her biting sense of humour. Especially when she says: "Mind you some days, I get my share of both."

"Not wearing deodorant, powder, or perfume, are you?" she asks.

"I read the brochure. I am au natural as ordered."

Handing me a gown, she says: "I can tell."

"Good, in view of what you are going to do to me, consider us even."

Laughing she says: "Remove all clothing from the waist up, and put on the gown."

She then leaves the room. A rather pointless nicety, considering I'll pull out what I'm hiding shortly.

She returns within seconds.

"Pull the gown off your left shoulder and place your left breast right here."

She points to the boob holder, which is a tray. Her request sounds easier than it is. Hello, I barely have breasts, how am I supposed to place nothing on a tray? It's absurdly difficult, but I manage to position my boob below the compression paddle, which lowers and applies pressure while taking low dose x-rays. Think of hands clapping in an up and down motion. Not displaying favouritism, she does the same to the right breast. Despite what I heard, it's painless. She says goodbye, instructs me to have a nice day, and hurries to meet her next boob. Left standing, I shed the gown, redress, and leave the office. Given I'm down-town, I decide to pick up my husband to save him a bus ride home.

I promised to call him when I'm done. Since I don't have a cell phone, I've borrowed my son's. Maybe, I'm odd. But I don't want to be reachable twenty-four seven. If you make yourself too available, people get mad when they can't contact you. I like a landline because I can de-cline to answer it, and excuses such as — "I guess I was outside" — are still plausible. The downside of my refusal to be a part of this century: Technology is advancing and I'm not. I take pictures of the lobby floor, call a few of my son's friends, and hope they don't see me as a crazy old lady who can't use a phone. With any luck, they'll think I'm the much more fashionable cougar. Grr ... Yeah right, barf. I take the elevator back to the clinic and ask to borrow their phone. The shame ...

Fred (not his real name, I would never marry a man named Fred) is waiting for me when I pull up. His silver hair shimmers in the sun-shine. A bulging briefcase rests at his feet. He grabs the bag and hurries to the car.

"How was the test?"

"Alright."

"Did it hurt?"

I pull away from the curb. I pay more attention to the surrounding cars than to his question.

"Not at all," I mutter.

He checks his watch. "We should pick up something to eat," he says.

We settle on takeout since it's getting late: ten to five. Oh my God, I'm getting old. I like to eat my last meal before six. Is sitting at Denny's at four-thirty in the afternoon, with a coupon in hand, the next step?

"I gave you a coupon, young lady. You discounted it, didn't you? Show me where you took it off the bill."

Kill me now.

We decide on hamburgers, a real treat since I'm gluten intolerant and can only cheat a few times a week without paying for it. I will not explain what that means because it's gross.

Twenty minutes later, we leave the drive through. I went to the bathroom so I lost my driving privileges. I don't care since I see driving as nothing more than a mode of transportation. The sack warms my knees. The gold wrappers glitter, and the aroma from the fried food thrashes the doggy odour, which usually engulfs the car. As we turn into our driveway, my thoughts centre on my hamburger. The reward for sticking to my restrictive diet for most of the week. I like food. Especially the stuff I'm not supposed to eat. We hang our coats and set the table. We're hungry, but we aren't barbarians. We use plates, not wrappers. The answering machine's red light blinks spastically. I try to ignore it, but as always, curiosity gets the best of me. I play the message. It's the clinic.

"You have an appointment for an ultrasound at two o'clock tomorrow afternoon. Arrive fifteen minutes early. Do not wear talcum powder, deodorant, or perfume."

They don't ask. They command. In hindsight, I should have ignored the red light and enjoyed my hamburger first. Another test is definitely not a good sign. I turn to Fred, forget it, I cannot even pretend to be married to Fred. His name is Luke, and clever that I am, I say: "They weren't supposed to call back."

I understand the ropes. You go for a test. Once you leave the premises, you cease to exist. Follow-up calls are inconvenient, and a faux pas. Annoying your doctor by requesting the results of the examination is rude. Protocol insists you forget about it. Months later, during a sched-uled appointment, your doctor may, or may not, mention that you went for the examination, and the results are negative. Why did they call me? I didn't expect a call back, nor did I want one.

Like most men, Luke is not good at reading body language. When my face pales, and my knuckles turn white as I clutch the counter, he suspects I'm having worrisome thoughts.

"Don't read too much into it," he says, as he bites into his burger.

Right, given the state of our healthcare system, you don't get an appointment for a test the following day, unless they saw something, and it was not good. Expedience has become frightening.

I'm incapable of speech. Shocked doesn't explain how I feel. I sit down and tell myself it's a fatty tumour, or a cyst. My hamburger tastes like sawdust. Its odour, which made my mouth water moments before, causes my stomach to lurch. I take a bite. I can barely swallow. When my husband isn't looking, I give the burger to Cane, our black lab. He finishes it before it touches the floor.

I pick at my fries. Luke tries to be entertaining and I pretend to be entertained. As soon as the meal is over, the dog belches, and I rush to the computer and begin googling. The literature instantly emphasizes that an abnormal mammogram does not mean you have cancer. The abnormity could be a denser breast tissue, a cyst, or a harmless lump such as fibroadenoma. It repeatedly highlights how benign conditions comprise the majority of abnormal mammograms. Ultrasounds are routinely advised when the mammogram detects a suspicious area. For every 1,000 U.S. women screened about 7% (70) will be called back. Ten will be referred for a biopsy; the remaining sixty will be diagnosed with a benign condition. Of the ten referred for biopsy, 3.5 will have cancer and 6.5 will not. Of the 3.5 who have cancer, two will have a low stage cancer that will be effectively cured after treatment. Reassuring statistics in the light of day, but as night descends, and I try to sleep, I can only think of malignancy, and the fact that the lab called back within two hours of my mammogram. I silently repeat encouraging statistics, but it's pointless.

In the dark, colour appears in the form of a mint green coat. I'm thirteen when my mother buys me the most amazing coat a mother ever purchased for her child. Stylish, it looks plucked from a fashion magazine. It's a maxi, which is the opposite of a mini, so it covers from neck to toes. The buttons are large and shiny. The cuffs have clips that tighten to form ruffles. It's also non-refundable since the store is going out of business. My mother takes a chance, which is uncharacteristic of her. Since money is tight, we never risk wasting it.

When she holds it up, my eyes grow wide. I grab it from her hands and hurriedly try it on.

During the seventies women wear cone bras, and coats have darts. The coat fits, with the exception of the chest. If I bump into something, or hold an object tightly, the material will invert. It is rather problematic, and definitely not a good look. *Hey, here comes the kid with the inverted boobs.* Not the sort of attention one seeks.

Mom laughs. "It'll fit next year," she assures me.

I believe her. My body type is similar to my mother's. She is well endowed. I have the curvy hips and an ample bottom. Within a year, I'll surely blossom. She takes the coat and hangs it in the dark recesses of our hall closet.

The following spring, Mom takes the coat out of the closet. We lay it on the bed. Its buttons gleam gloriously. I touch the soft material and my pulse quickens. Mom holds it up. I rush over to try it on. My smile plummets as I tie the buttons. My mother's smile vanishes before I can tie the belt.

It still doesn't fit. Mom's reassuring words are not as encouraging. Back in the closet it goes.

By the third year, the coat has become a harbinger of spring. As soon as winter's hold loosens, the closet door opens, and voila, the coat emerges. I see it, and grimace. It's a test. I fail repeatedly.

We no longer smile. Nor do we comment on the coat's beauty. I try it on because I have to. It's now shorter — and tight across the shoulders. However the risk of implosion remains. Without uttering a word, Mom takes the coat, and hangs it back into the closet.

A day after the coat's annual outing, I'm walking to school. I see my cousin, four years my junior, walking ahead. Her gait is lively. She's wearing a new coat, and looks proud. It is mint green and has very large shiny buttons, and cuffs that create ruffles above her wrists. She spins around and the coat forms a magnificent arc. Sandy sees me; smiles, and waves excitedly. I pretend not to see her, turn the corner, and slow my step.

I hate mint green to this very day. It reminds me of breasts that obstinately refused to grow. If one of them grew a tumour, I swear I'll rip it off myself.

Stupid breasts, stupid mammograms.

2

Y FAMILIARITY WITH ultrasounds involves seeing my unborn children. I smile and nod, feigning understanding whenever the technician points at an appendage, and believe *I'm having a well-endowed boy, instead of a girl with a set of arms and legs.* I'm confused, but the experience is decidedly more joyous than looking for a tumour. How does the scenario go when it's a tumour? Do they point out their observations?

Oh look it's round and self-contained — fatty, fatty, two by four, guess you don't go to the oncology ward.

See all those spikes and the irregular shape — Spiky, spiky, oh that is bad. You have cancer, oh so sad.

The technician performing the ultrasound is polite and professional, and has the demeanour of an undertaker. This test is no joking matter. But let's pretend I have a chance of living long enough to leave the room.

My memory of the thousands of dollars spent on research — proving how laughter decreases pain, boosts immunity, lowers stress hormones, eases fear, and anxiety — must be faulty. For whenever you face a medical emergency, those around you often look as if they lost their best friend. Do you not want to save us? Admit it: you spent the money figuring out ways of ridding the system of the sick. It's a Machiavellian budget scheme, isn't it?

Or is your long face an attempt to appear sensitive? *This woman is having a test done to look for a cancerous tumour. Show her grief, show her sombreness, and look as if you're dying too.* Do they honestly think that makes things better? You might as well hire a hole-digger to sit in the waiting room. Ravens at the front desk would be a nice touch. I admit I sometimes look at things differently, but comedians should be at the front line of our health care system. That way, even if the treatment is unsuccessful, you'll leave this world laughing, and one minute of laughter is worth more than an hour of anxiety.

Recumbent on the table, I can't muster a complaint as she applies the cold sticky gel to my right breast. It's the obvious troublemaker.

Gel makes the breast slippery so a small transducer, a device that picks up sound waves, can slide along the skin, sending waves through it. The principle is the same as the sonar used by bats. When a sound wave strikes an object, it bounces back. By measuring echo waves it's possible to ascertain how far away the object is, and its shape, size and consistency (whether the mass is solid or filled with fluid).

"What made you have a mammogram?" the woman asks, without taking her eyes off the screen in front of her.

The image has become so important she can't take a second to glance in my direction. Does she not know niceties go a long way? A smile, a nod, a quick peek, any of those things, would make me feel like an individual, instead of a potentially cancerous boob. I swallow bitter feelings.

"I thought I felt something a few months ago, but it went away. I assumed it was a cyst. When I went to my doctor, she didn't feel anything, but she suggested I have the test since I am fifty. Since I've had the mammogram, I can now feel a tiny lump."

"Show me," she says.

I place my finger just above my nipple. She informs me it is at the twelve o'clock position. I never knew that breasts are read like clocks. My lump is sitting on the stroke of midnight. She begins to slide the transducer over my right breast. She focuses on where I told her I could feel the lump.

"That's odd," she mutters, and I feel my first pang of apprehension. "So you didn't feel an unvarying lump?" she asks. I don't like the incredulity ringing in her voice. I also don't appreciate how she refuses to look me in the eyes.

"On occasion but usually not," I explain. Apprehension turns to dread. She doesn't read me as well as I can read her. She shakes her head, and I shiver.

Dammit, she should know most people can read head shakes! They are never complimentary. They usually signify disappointment, and sometimes, especially if eye rolling is involved, they denote exasperation. I didn't see her roll her eyes, but I suspect she did.

Dimwit, why didn't you come for testing earlier? Don't you recognize cancer, you stupid twit?

Oh my god, I have cancer and, as an added bonus, I'm a tad stupid.

It's over. She moves away from the screen, and stands up, without saying a word. She begins to retreat.

"Get dressed. Your doctor will have the results in a week."

I whisper goodbye, but she has already left the room. I'm alone with air that feels heavy and dark. I tell myself I'm being paranoid. The only problem is I'm not prone to paranoia. I failed the damn test. I know I did.

The experience leaves me vulnerable. I deserve a treat. I stop off at the grocery store and buy a loaf of French bread. I indulge in two crispy toasts before I put the bread away. I now have a stomach-ache and most likely a cancerous breast. All in all, not a good day.

*J*T TURNS OUT I'm not the only one having an ultrasound. My niece, Caitlin, finds out she's pregnant. The youngest family member is thirteen, so the prospect of fresh blood elicits excitement.

As a child, Caitlin had the longest, skinniest legs and arms of anyone I knew. When angered, limbs flew in every direction. Would her child be the same? Would his or her tantrums encompass a whole room? Considering Caitlin is five-seven, and her husband is six-foot-five, I envision the child having the capacity to touch all four nursery walls at once.

9-1-1 please help us. We cannot reach the baby; his foot is jamming the door.

You mean he's in front of the door and you're afraid to open it.

No the baby is in the crib, but he's stretching, and we're worried we'll break his leg if we force the door open.

I love babies. I'll carry him or her, even if his or her legs touch my knees.

When I visit my husband's family, everyone speaks of the new mother and the progress of her pregnancy. Something is growing within her, and it's beautiful and revitalizing. Something is growing inside of me, but it's hideous and deadly. Caitlin shares her experience. She talks of ultrasounds, and weight gains. Her tone denotes excitement and anticipation. She revels in her body's ability to produce new life.

I hide my experience. I hope it'll dissipate into groundless fear. Caitlin's situation is so different from mine it counterbalances my despair and brings hope. Not everything in this world is bad. A point I recently often remind myself of, because the big C is about chaos, confusion, and catastrophe.

Textbooks describe cancer as a malignant tumour or growth, caused when cells multiply uncontrollably, destroying healthy tissue. Researchers give no mention to the consumption of healthy thoughts, and the birth of destructive, negative feelings. Even the very threat of cancer will not allow you to disregard it. Bursting into your consciousness, like its concrete form, thoughts multiply uncontrollably.

Everything is going to change. You're not normal. You're sick. Malignancy. Have you noticed it has your name in it? Do you know what malign means? It denotes evil and wrongdoing. It's hurtful. Something bad is out to hurt you.

Say goodbye to your breast. Maybe even your life. Your plans for the future? Kaput. You don't have a future. Unless you think dying of an agonizing disease is a future. The strength you imagine you possess will buckle, as will you, as you fall to the floor and beg death to take you.

Fuck off eh!

"I'm cancelling the trip," my husband says as we tidy the kitchen after dinner.

I clean the counter mechanically.

"Don't be silly. You'll be back in three days. You planned the conference months ago. Just go. I'm sure it's nothing. I'm fine."

When he gives me a worried look, I ramble on about statistics. As his forehead relaxes, I know he's feeling reassured.

I'm lying. Nonetheless, I convince him to go. I thrust the dread deep inside of me, until it is a tinny voice, off in the distance.

My children say I hate to be wrong about anything. They're mistaken. I want my perceptions to be false. I want to be reading things that are not there. My little bump is a cyst. I'm blowing everything out of proportion. I'm guilty of the classic mistake: Making a mountain out of a molehill. I can live with being foolish. I want my life to revert to normal. I don't want to be the woman with cancer.

When Luke leaves for the conference, I feel triumphant. The hard lump does not have the power to change how I live. Sometimes you must make a molehill out of a mountain. It's the only way to get beyond it.

OCTOBER 7, A warm day, a sunny day, my mother's birthday. I open my eyes and know with absolute certainty: news is coming my way. My stomach churns; bubbles of fear make it choppy. The report will not be good.

Premonitions aren't strangers. I don't turn my back on them. If I push them out of my way, a rude shock smacks me from behind.

I'm an only child. My mother's birthday will continue as planned. Cancer won't be my world. It might take a part of me, but I refuse to let it take all of me. Life has to go on. Mom knows nothing of the tests I've had, and she isn't going to, until the diagnosis is firm and unavoidable.

The day begins with a butterfly exhibition. Within a humid greenhouse, hundreds of butterflies flit from flower to flower. Most are species I've never seen before, even though they're indigenous. Hands hold slices of oranges, in hopes of attracting the fluttering creatures. Butterflies, like humans, soon tire of excess, and ignore the extended arms. All of God's creatures appreciate what's gone, what's no longer offered.

My mother stands perfectly still. A brown butterfly lands on the orange slice she holds. Black orbs decorate the papery surface. They look like gems. Mom admires the delicateness of the butterflies, and the array of colours that paint their wings. I admire their strength. Imagine, a weightless creature battling the elements, to migrate thousands of miles every year. It's seemingly impossible. Inspiring.

Once we leave the show, we stop for a quick lunch and then go antiquing. Okay, I'm being intentionally vague, outright lying to be exact. We go to second hand shops. I love those stores. You feel Trumped as you glance through their wares. Whatever they have, you can afford.

What will you find? You never know, and that's the fun of it. Mom buys a silver chain with a teardrop amber pendant dangling delicately. I find an oriental umbrella stand in shades of brown, red, and gold. Hand painted and superbly detailed. I never use umbrellas. But that doesn't prevent it from being a steal — only thirty-five dollars!

Last stop is dinner at home. I'm making mom's favourite: tacos. It seems like an odd choice for a birthday celebration, but when you live alone, you don't buy foods that come in boxes of twelve portions.

It's a small celebration. My mother is a widow, my son is working, and Luke is out of town. So the party consists of my daughter Madison, my mom, and me. Just as I crunch the last morsel of taco on my plate, the phone peals. I snatch it, and hurry from the room. My doctor's voice does not faze me. I knew who it was even before I picked up the handset. I make my way down the stairs to the basement. From the start, I hide cancer in deep dark recesses.

The first words out of her mouth are: "Don't become alarmed."

I become alarmed.

"They did find a mass and further investigation is warranted. Don't assume the worst. I've forwarded the results from your ultrasound to the Breast Health Clinic. They'll schedule you for a procedure called a core biopsy. After taking samples of the lump, they'll send it to a pathologist, who'll then determine what we're dealing with."

"You mean if it's benign or cancerous?"

"Yes, but don't upset yourself yet. It can be many things other than cancer. The Breast Clinic is very good at what they do. They should call you within a few days, and tell you when the procedure will take place. If they don't, call them. Here's the number."

I grab a pen and paper. My hand trembles as I write down the number. We say our goodbyes and I hurry back to the birthday celebration. Madison clears the dishes, as she and my mother chat about her new job. I find a lighter and set aglow the candles on the coffee cake I made the night before. Mom smiles when I place it in front of her. Her favourite — sour cream coffee cake with a crispy coating of brown sugar and cinnamon.

"Make a wish," I say, with all the gaiety I can muster.

My mother's cheeks puff out. She leans over the cake and blows with all her might. Smoke wafts from all the candles.

Madison begins to sing *Happy Birthday* and I join in. We sing like bullfrogs, who in turn sound like the yelp of a broken guitar string. After we butcher the song, I cut each of us a slice of cake.

Madison, like me, is gluten intolerant. We tell each other we must have cake. It's a birthday celebration and eating birthday cake is mandatory. We're both liars. We eat cake because we love cake, cookies, and all the other things our bodies can't digest. The cake lies trapped on a fancy platter. We attack it like locusts. Mom has one piece, and wipes her mouth delicately with a birthday napkin when done.

It's now time to open gifts. My mother grew up during the depression. She unties ribbons, and removes the wrapping paper without ripping it. I'm impatient. I always want to grab the present from her hands and tear the paper off.

Like all loving mothers, she proclaims: "You shouldn't have bought so much."

The night winds down. Chatter becomes weary. I'm surprised neither of them thought to ask me who called. If they had, I would have lied. The evening ends quietly, without fanfare.

$\mathcal{M}$Y CANCER IS a pushy little bugger. From the beginning, it manages to intrude on all of our celebrations. First, my mother's birthday, and now beside the turkey on Thanksgiving. I'm the only one who sees it. Nonetheless, it's real. We invite thirteen people to share the holiday. An uninvited guest aims to take centre stage. Every time I enter the room with another dish, it leaps in front of the plate, before I can set it down. I pretend not to see it, doing the tasks one expects from a host, albeit with shaky hands.

Cancer has become my embarrassing relative. You know, the one that enters a room, and causes everyone's eyes to seek one another's, in a quiet yet tangible: "Oh shit, I can't believe they showed up, the nerve!"

Every family has the cretin who innately says and does the wrong thing. They can't help themselves. It's their nature. Even quiet and stationary, their very presence causes discomfort. I brought the miscreant to the table. I sit and it peers at me menacingly. I have a choice. I can ignore it, or force everyone to see it.

I look around the table at the faces of those I love. What would they say if I tell them what I'm going through? I can find out. The truth could easily spill from my lips, since it never leaves my head.

Pass the cranberries. By the way, I'm being tested for breast cancer and it doesn't look good.

Would the plate fall? Would anyone pick it up? I'm not ready to find out. I want to pretend to be like everyone else. We're all healthy. We complain about silly things, never realizing how trivial our complaints are. I refuse to welcome the albatross into the room. Today is turkey day!

I toss the albatross outside. It circles overhead, without tiring. I laugh heartily and join the conversations that drift across the table. My mother's stuffing looks plump and flavourful in a festive orange bowl. I place two heaping scoops on my plate. If I'm going to battle cancer, I'm not going to chew on carrots. No sirree. Screw the albatross, screw gluten. Pass the cherry pie.

*D*AYS PASS. THE clinic doesn't call. I find myself staring at the phone. Its stillness feels like a slight.

The request to come in for an ultrasound, hours after the mammogram, terrified me. Silence now panics me. What's happening? I was never the type to worry, let alone feel fear. I should be relieved that a rapid summons is not forthcoming. It has to be a good sign.

I don't buy it. The mass in my breast may be cancer. Why am I dangling from a pink ribbon? It's a cruel torture.

Making matters worse, October is Breast Cancer month. Everywhere I go I see pink ribbons. Every store I frequent asks for donations. The television runs commercials for finding the cure. I may not have noticed if I didn't have a mass sitting inside my breast but I do and all the attention is a constant reminder.

I'm grateful the funding for breast cancer is substantial, yet I want everyone to back off. Quit asking for money. Quit showing me survivors. Quit explaining the disease to me. Just quit ... The pink ribbon becomes a noose. I don't want to be one of their statistics.

I'm in a bad place. I always hate waiting. Usually I feel impatient and put out. This time I'm fearful. I almost call the number my doctor gave me for the clinic. I talk myself out of it. Asking for things goes against my nature. I sit back and wait. I'm ridiculously polite. I don't like to appear pushy or arrogant. (Two attributes I keep in check.) Many people are waiting for calls. We all have to wait our turn, regardless of how nerve wrenching it is.

Days pass. It's now over a week. Angry, I call the number. It's no longer in service. I look the number up in the phonebook. It connects me to a computerized service that gives you oodles of choices for doctors, but I don't have the name of a doctor, so it doesn't do me any good.

When I call my family physician, a machine informs me the receptionist is away from her desk, and I will have to call again. I try for hours. My only accomplishment is a sweaty ear and cramped fingers.

The receptionist is never at her desk. It takes me two days to reach a human being.

"Doctor Fungus' office, how may I help you?"

"Hello I'm Nancy Burns. I'm calling because ..." And I explain. "I was wondering if you could give me the correct number, and tell me whom I should ask for." The line is silent. "She told me to call if I hadn't heard anything within a few days, and it has been over a week."

The voice speaks with authority. "You are not Doctor Fungus' patient. You are Doctor You Should Have Picked Me's patient."

I hear ringing for another line, before I can argue the fact.

"Doctor You Should Have Picked Me's office, how may I help you?"

"Hi, I'm Nancy Burns. I'm Doctor Fungus' patient. I explained this to her receptionist but I was transferred to you."

The pinging of buttons volleys me back to Fungus' receptionist, the newly christened Miss Maggot.

"Hello, you have reached Dr. Fungus' office. How may I help you?"

"Hello, this is Nancy Burns. I was speaking to you before you transferred me to another doctor. Believe me, I'm a patient of Doctor Fungus. I've been seeing her for twenty years."

"No you're not her patient. You're Doctor You Should Have Picked Me's patient."

I find an accurate measure of stupidity is how dim-witted a person can believe someone else is. This woman is off the chart.

"I'm not Doctor You Should Have Picked Me's patient. I have never even met the man. I know my doctor, and it is Doctor Fungus."

"The computer says that you're Doctor You Should Have Picked Me's patient."

We created technology to enable, not disable. If it bears the burden of judgment, you're too dependent. I lost it. How can someone believe I don't know the name of my own doctor? Did I not just say I'd been seeing her for twenty years?

"I don't care what your computer says; I'm Doctor Fungus' patient. Your computer is wrong."

"What is your name again?"

"Nancy-Gail Burns," I declare through clenched teeth. I can feel myself become snarly and snappish. My life is at the mercy of fools!

"Nancy-Gail Burns is a patient of Doctor Fungus, but Nancy Burns is Doctor You Should Have Picked Me's patient."

By now, I know there's no point in arguing. I once again explain how I need the phone number of the Breast Health Clinic, and perhaps my file can tell her the name of the doctor who's suppose to call me.

"I don't know what you're talking about," Maggot says, yawning.

Frustrated, I huff: "Perhaps Doctor Fungus can call me. I'm waiting for an appointment for a biopsy, to find out if I have cancer. It's rather important."

"The doctor is too busy to call patients."

I feel thrown into a comedy routine that's not funny in the least.

"Perhaps you can look in my file and find the number of the Breast Health Clinic. Doctor Fungus sent the results of my ultrasound to them, and they were supposed to call me. If you could find the number, I'll call myself."

By this point, I'm nearly begging.

I hear shuffling. She comes back on the line.

"This is the number but don't call them today. Wait until tomorrow."

I call the clinic as soon as I hang up.

"Hello, Breast Health Clinic, how may I help you?"

"I'm Nancy Burns. I'm calling to find out when my appointment for a core biopsy is."

The nurse finds my name in their computer and laughs.

"I just received the fax a moment ago. You don't waste any time, do you?"

"What do you mean a moment ago? My doctor sent you the ultrasound results over a week ago."

Keys click. "No, we just got it."

"I received a call from the doctor on October seventh. She said she sent the results, and I would hear from you within a few days."

"We contact people within a day of receiving the results. We have no record of you, other than the fax sent minutes ago." I'm speechless. "You mean you've been waiting all that time to hear from us. You must be so worried."

She has a soft voice, full of compassion.

"I was wondering why no one called me."

"Sorry dear, but we didn't even know about you until today. We wouldn't make you wait that long. I can imagine what you've been thinking. Give me fifteen minutes to check our schedule. I'll call you back as soon as I have an appointment for you."

The telephone rings ten minutes later. "How about next Wednesday?"

"That would be perfect."

"I'm sorry about the wait."

"No need to be. Five days isn't very long."

"Is ten good for you?"

"Ten is fine."

I call Fungus' office.

"I would like to make an appointment to see the doctor?"

"Her calendar is full," Maggot informs me. "She can see you next month."

"What about walk-in hours."

"Walk-in hours are Friday, nine until noon."

I hang up. I'll be in Fungus' waiting room by nine. I'm furious. I've been waiting for a call that would never have come, if I hadn't spoken to Fungus' receptionist. Maggot knew the ultrasound results were never sent. She faxed them as I was speaking to her. She didn't want me to call the clinic because she knew they would tell me they just received them. I foolishly think my doctor will be outraged by what has taken place.

On Friday, I march into the doctor's office, clutching my bag of indignation. I'm grateful not to see patients filling the waiting room. This won't take long.

"Nancy Burns. I'm here to see the doctor."

"The doctor is not in."

I recognize Maggot's voice. "Two days ago you told me Friday mornings are for walk ins."

She looks up at me and rolls her eyes. "They are, but not this week."

"It didn't occur to you to tell me that on Wednesday."

She is giving me only half her attention, as she looks down at papers and shuffles them.

"The doctor is on holidays."

Her tone suggests I'm the only person in the northern hemisphere who doesn't know that. I guess I didn't receive the international bulletin.

"When is she back?" I ask through clenched lips.

"The doctor will be in on Monday."

"I'd like an appointment."

"Her appointment book is full. She can't see you Monday."

"Okay Tuesday."

"Tuesday is busy too."

"Listen here. This is an emergency. I have to see the doctor."

I can hear haughtiness ring in my voice. It would usually embarrass me, but when someone gives no thought to your safety, you have to spring forth with all your might.

Maggot honours me with a look reserved for unreasonable assholes. I don't care. I hold her stare. I give her the best stink eyes I can conjure. My eyes are so brown they appear black. I am the master of stink eyes. She drops her gaze first.

"I can give you an appointment for noon on Tuesday, but she will only give you ten minutes." (I think it is the slot reserved for unreasonable assholes.)

"Fine, I'll take it."

Outrage replaces my desire to appear reasonable. I don't deserve this kind of treatment. No one does. Health care is a right, not a privilege. I've been Fungus' patient for over twenty years. A test will confirm whether my suspicious lump is cancerous. A test I had wrongly assumed was booked days previously. I want to talk to my doctor. Is that too much to ask?

7

*J*T IS A quarter to twelve. The waiting room looks like a convention hall for individuals attending anger management. People stand with their backs against the wall, glaring. Children cry, and whine. Sighs fill the air as glances check watches.

At one-thirty, I hear my name.

Maggot leads the way down a long hallway. I silently rehearse what I'm going to say. I don't want to babble. I'll give her the facts, and let her do what she wants with them.

Instead of an examination room, Maggot leads me to Fungus' office. I sit in a hard backed chair and look at posters, illustrating diseases. I learn about prostate cancer, maladies of the eye, and I've just about memorized the parts of the reproductive system when the doctor casually breezes in. A few more minutes and I would have been ready to take the entrance exam for medical school.

Fungus' brown curls discharge in every direction. Her lab coat looks crumpled.

"I don't understand the mix-up. I sent the fax on October the seventh, just as I told you."

Her receptionist obviously told her the story, and she's taking responsibility for the fax the clinic never received. I had wrongly assumed Maggot had sent the original fax.

"It never arrived," I reply calmly.

Prepared, she pulls out a dated confirmation of the fax. The paper flies across my vision line in a blur.

"As you can see, I sent it and I have a confirmation that they received it."

Her voice is icy. I nod, rather than admit to seeing nothing, but seriously, an action hero with super powers would have had difficulty reading it.

She continues to blame the clinic, while I think back on all the problems I've had with her in the past. This is not the first time test results were lost in limbo, and it's always someone else's fault. Never having been seriously ill, I repeatedly ignored her shortcomings. The competence of your doctor is rarely questioned when you're healthy.

Regardless of the error's architect, her defensive attitude wears thin. It never occurs to her to say: "Waiting must have been nerve-wracking. Luckily, you called the office. I'm so sorry for the mix-up."

"You told me to call the clinic, if they didn't call me, and the number you gave me is defunct. Furthermore, it took me two days to get through to your receptionist. I was constantly told she was away from her desk and to call back."

"We were on holidays. She must have forgotten to change the message."

"I spent hours calling."

"Other people have complained. I've told her to be more vigilant."

Once again, no apology is forthcoming.

"When I asked her if you could call me, she said you're too busy to call patients."

Before I can say more, she cuts me off.

"May I speak," she says in a self-important voice. "You have to understand a doctor's schedule. We can't return every message we receive." (Not even from a person who may have cancer?) She stares into my eyes and says: "Do you know my work schedule? I arrive early in the morning, and I leave late at night. I'm sure she tacked the message on my board, and it fell off before I could read it."

I'm confused. Is she too harried to call patients? Or does her message system consist of notes tacked on a bulletin board? If it hadn't fallen off, would she have called me? I'm at a loss on how to respond. I feel she is greedy and has too many patients if she doesn't have time to return a call from a person facing a serious illness. As for the bulletin board, you must be kidding. If messages routinely fall off, and you do not update your system, what does that say about you and your relationship with your patients?

She talks about a doctor's schedule, acting as if her education negates her responsibility to be a decent person. She has sworn to help others, yet when she dons the white coat, she strips herself of the everyday clothing all of us wear. A doctor should put their lab coat over their clothing. It should be an addition to their character, not a subtraction.

Doctor Fungus and I shared a long relationship. Before my threat of cancer, I never asked her to call me. When I reach out, in a time of need, I discover I'm not deserving of her compassion, or precious time. My body tightens in anger, and then slumps in despair. I'm only beginning my journey into illness. The coldness I encounter chills me to my core.

Jumping on my silence, she fills it with hypocrisy.

"You must realize that we're worried about you. I spoke with my receptionist and we're appalled that the fax didn't go through like it was supposed to."

She makes no mention of being appalled at the hours I spent trying to reach her, when she was not even in the office.

"She couldn't have been too worried since she didn't even know who I was," I say, "and tried to convince me that I was Doctor You Should Have Picked Me's patient."

"English is not her first language. Maybe I shouldn't have her manning the front desk."

Do ya think? Doctor Fungus then proceeds to act indignant.

"Here are the copies of your tests," she barks, as she thrusts papers at me. Insulted she leaves the office without looking at me. The door slams, the wall shudders. I'm left sitting there, wondering how she can walk away without apologizing, or at least wishing me luck. I have a feeling if I call her office next week, Maggot will answer my call. In my doctor's mind, I did something wrong. How rude of me to complain about missing tests, and really the audacity of mentioning how two days of my life was wasted phoning people who weren't even in the office. I criticized her, the nerve!

I return to my car and read the results of my ultrasound. They are cold and clinical. I become detached from the person they're describing.

Right Breast Ultrasound
The patient is 50 years old and has no significant risk factors for breast carcinoma. The examination is compared to bilateral mammography from Oct 1, 2009. At 12:00 o'clock where a lump is noted, a 20 × 11 × 12mm hypocchoic, ill defined solid mass is

seen, which is highly suspicious for breast carcinoma. This lesion represents the speculated nodular opacity described on mammography. No other solid or cystic lesion seen within the right breast. There is at least one lymph node of the right axilla, measuring 26 × 13 × 13mm. Percutaneous biopsy under ultrasound guidance is recommended, as well as consultation in general surgery. Report was faxed to Doctor's office on 2–10–09.

Fungus called me on the seventh, supposedly sent a fax to the clinic, and promptly forgot about it.

I believed general practitioners were navigators who helped patients plot a course through an illness. Plunged into the land of sickness, the familiar face I relied on is gone. I'll enter the world of oncologists, invasive tests, and alien medical lingo alone.

I start the car and drive home on autopilot. Once home I hide the papers in my underwear drawer. The test results are filthy, and I don't want anyone to see them. Later that night, I sneak into the drawer and pluck them out of the wads of undergarments. In the privacy of my bathroom, I examine them. Read them twice. Return them to their hiding place. Step into the tub. Within seconds, sweat forms on my brow. Dizziness causes my vision to blur. I run to the toilet and throw up my dinner.

Nooooo!!!!!

At the time, I didn't know anything about the Breast Imaging-Reporting and Data system (BI-RADS). After my bath, I fire up the computer. I find out what I need to know.

Mammogram results are expressed in terms of the BI-RADS Assessment Category, often called a BI-RADS score. The categories range from zero to six. The Assessment Categories are:

- 0: Incomplete
- 1: Negative
- 2: Benign finding(s)
- 3: Probably benign
- 4: Suspicious abnormality
- 5: Highly suggestive of malignancy
- 6: Known biopsy — proven malignancy

Highly suggestive of malignancy was not the description used by the woman who did the ultrasound! It's the description used by all technicians to classify a mass into category five. Category 5 means the lesion has a ninety-five percent probability of being malignant. The only higher category is a six. It's used when the lesion is known to be malignant. I can see why my doctor of twenty years isn't concerned. The report doesn't have her name on it. Some will say such an accusation is mean spirited, but how else can you classify her actions?

My summation doesn't please me. I gave my trust to a woman for twenty years, only to find out I was a fool.

I'll never see her again. I'll visit clinics, and receive treatment from strangers. If they don't care, you can't blame them.

Fungus taught me a lesson. Don't put your health in someone else's hands. Illness is not a passive sport. Learn all you can about your opponent, rely on your team, but remember, it's ultimately your battle.

8

SYNONYMS FOR *PATIENT* are:

> *tolerant*
> *long suffering*
> *accepting*
> *even tempered*
> *submissive*

My worst character traits are:

> *intolerant*
> *impatient*
> *defiant*
> *short-tempered*
> *challenging*

If I had to apply for the job of patient, I wouldn't get the position.

Sorry there must have been some sort of mistake. The candidate you're seeking isn't me. This obviously won't work out.

～○

Powerless, I seek power.

When you enter the world of traditional medicine, strangers become warriors, plied against your adversary. You don't know these people, but your life is in their hands. You trust their skills will save you. You have to, or the battle is lost from the onset.

Tests, which are beneficial, necessary, and life saving, are dual natured. They are also invasive, frightening and sometimes painful. I'm thankful for the advancements made, but also overwhelmed.

I cannot, will not, dismiss the influence of my own mind. My life is at stake. I have to be an active participant in the battle taking place. To do less would mean I'm a failure to myself.

The brain is the commander of the craft. Presently my body is in a state of mutiny. It has turned upon itself. I must seize control.

I grab hold of the reins. My mind can accomplish amazing feats. Positive thinking and visualization can coexist with western medicine. Think placebo effect: If you tell yourself you're feeling better, you often do feel better.

Whenever I take a bath, I gaze down at my breast. It looks the same, but I look at it differently. It is no longer familiar and trustworthy. The breast I knew so well is gone. In its place is a vessel that holds a trespasser, intent on pillaging my body.

I give my enemy a name and a concrete imaginary form. I prepare for battle. Spike, my cancer, is a crazy little terrier who is out of control. Snarly and vicious, you dare not turn your back on him. Instead, you face him head on, and order him to obey.

I don't think my visual imagery will make the cancer disappear. I do believe it can restrain Spike, put him on a leash, so to speak.

Fine you are sitting in my breast. You entered through an open gate, and you wandered onto my property. I accept that.

I recognize you for what you are. You're a bad dog. You're one of the cruellest of predators. You have no mercy. Well, neither will I.

I will leash you. I will not feed you. You expect me to cower in fear. I will not. I will not play dead. I will impose that role on you.

Foisted on me, you will live by my rules. You're an unruly little beast. I will force you to sit and stay. You will not be free to roam and do as you please.

I spend hours holding Spike. My hand cups him, keeps him small and, most importantly of all, keeps him sedentary. His eyes dart. I can see his mind working. He wants to bolt. I yank the leash until it is short and taut. Spike is not having control of the yard. He will sit on the stroke of midnight and never see daybreak.

I'm not the ideal patient, but I'm determined, pushy, and tenacious. *Watch your back, Spike. You've met your match.*

9

*T*HE MORNING IS cold, sunny, and bright. Vestiges of fall cling to the day. Fallen leaves are slick. Strides are precarious. Bodies stiffen against the onslaught of the sudden chill. Winter is coming and he appears nasty.

The biopsy is today. Only Luke, and my best friend, Judy, know I'm having it done. It's a secret. Is having cancer a sin? In a way it is. If I have cancer, I have not sinned. The cancer itself is sinful. Cancer hurts. Cancer scares. Cancer palls life with its touch. Only when the diagnosis is firm will I tell my adult children. The same rules apply to my mother, who lives alone. I don't want her sitting with my cancer as company. Cancer might have me in its grip. But let them be free for a little longer.

Luke wants to accompany me.

"It's not necessary," I say, as I dress for the day, choosing my clothes carefully. Sad days necessitate effort.

"You shouldn't go alone."

I turn and glare. "Why not? I'm an adult and it's a small procedure."

"But —"

"I don't need to have my hand held."

His eyes hold hurt. I turn away. I can't give credence to the reality of cancer. I don't want to be sick, nor do I want to need people. The thought of losing my autonomy terrifies me.

Grief has five stages — so the story goes. I straddle the denial fence, and falter between accepting cancer, and denying what it entails. Cancer and illness don't co-exist in my mind. Being outwardly healthy makes the delusion easier.

Judy insists I drive to her house after the test. Positive it's a fatty tumour, she believes the biopsy will rid our world of malignancy.

The Breast Health Clinic is a separate building from the hospital. Unsure of its exact location, I follow a woman wearing the telltale pink zippy with the ribbon logo. My powers of deduction are greater than my sense of direction. I find the clinic without mishap.

Arriving fifteen minutes before my appointment, I glance at the books filling the waiting room. Most are about breast cancer and plastic surgery, but typical women's magazines also litter the tables. I refuse to be anxious, and try to convince myself I don't belong. Cognitively I sense I have cancer, but emotionally ... no, no, no, not going there until I have to.

I focus on the five percent chance of it being a horrible mistake. My hand grabs a copy of *House and Home*. I don't give a damn about stylish homes and decorating tips. I peer over the magazine and look around. Many women are waiting. Most have ill at ease men sitting beside them. The majority are older white women, but there are a few of different age and ethnic groups. A veiled Muslim woman has three young children with her. She spends her time keeping them quiet.

Will she find herself in the elite group of newly diagnosed cancer patients? Eighty percent of breast cancer occurs in woman over fifty. However, there are still twenty percent of women diagnosed much younger. Will the three young children reach out to find no mother's hand to grasp theirs?

I could be one of the statistics that fall outside of the norm too. The thought is unsettling, surreal. The line between healthy and unhealthy suddenly seems nonexistent. I don't want to cross over the line. I want to stay where I am. I don't like to travel.

The faces around me appear shell-shocked. Are they wondering: "Why me? What am I doing here?" Does anyone ask: "Why shouldn't it be me? We believe tragedy should strike faceless strangers. Yet every face is familiar, and treasured by someone.

I sit in the pink waiting room, and look at the people who fill the rows of chairs. The Muslim woman chases her young son. Her foot catches in her long dress. Just as she's about to fall, she rights herself. I hope that she'll remain safe. Since she isn't white, and Caucasians have the highest incidence of breast cancer, she has one factor in her favour.

When they call my name, I rise. A woman leads me down the corridor to a group of change rooms and lockers. I'm told to remove all clothing from the waist up and to wear two one-size-fits-all gowns. (They actually fit no one. I think a monk from the Spanish Inquisition designed them for the sheer hell of it). The first ties in the back, the second ties in the front. It is a pseudo nightgown and housecoat.

They're well worn and frequently laundered. How many women have worn the gown? Were they scared? Brave? Numb? A mixture of all three? Can you wash emotions from a garment? Or is the softness of the material, their touch? Their well wishes?

The johnnies are too big and I'm constantly rearranging them. I see the pink zippy woman waiting in the small anteroom. She wears gowns that match my own. When I sit down beside her, we smile at one another. We immediately know each other's situation. She has gone through what I'm just beginning. That's why she wears the survivor's zippy.

"First time here?" she asks.

"Yeah, I'm scheduled for a biopsy."

My answer causes her lips to purse. "It's not that bad," she assures me, but her facial expression doesn't back up her words.

They call her name before we can say anything more. I see her leave as I'm following the nurse into the biopsy room. She touches the leg of the woman who had been sitting next to me. I hadn't spoken to her because she was reading a paperback book, and didn't seem to want to talk.

"I got another year," she whispers in a melancholy voice.

The woman doesn't say anything. She smiles, but it is puny. I don't understand their interaction. Everything went well but they're not joyful. I'm a neophyte who doesn't understand. Reoccurrences can take place years after the initial treatment. A good year is only that.

I lie down on the examination table. The ultrasound machine, parked next to the bed, is inches from my head. It'll guide the biopsy. I try to watch the console as the technician zooms into my underarm, but its closeness makes it impossible to see. Only a moment passes before the radiologist is called. They confer. The first ultrasound report mentioned the size of one node. It must be larger than it's supposed to be. Can a node be fat? Or is cancer wrapped around it? They are conversing at my feet. I overhear everything they say. They conclude the node is normal. Had it been abnormal, would they have parleyed in hushed tones?

Normal, average, such insulting words unless you are facing abnormal and atypical. There are moments when you don't want to stand out from the crowd. I feel my first flow of gratitude. It's a good sign.

The mass might be cancerous but it appears as though it hasn't spread to the nodes. Spike is sitting still. Good bad dog.

The biopsy is about to begin. They give me something to freeze the site.

"You'll feel pressure but no pain," the technician says. "We'll take three to six samples." She shows me the device they'll be using and fires it in the air so I can hear its abrupt, ringing sound. It reminds me of my staple gun, the one I use to re-upholster furniture.

Aptly referred to as a biopsy gun, some women take offense to the term. Pointing a gun at a woman's breast is a faux pas. Bickering over terminology is ridiculous. It is what it is. It fires into your breast and seizes a sample. It doesn't sound nice, because it isn't nice. Changing the name will not change the experience.

I lie on my back. The ties of the gown are undone. My right breast is exposed. My right arm is over my head. I wait for it to begin. As an adult, I understand the concept of the greater good. Private, I despise being exposed and touched. Health care workers strip personal space and modesty from you. Liberties you would never permit are an integral part of the treatment. Months later, a nurse will tell me to leave modesty at the door. Even at the onset, I knew I was better off boxing it and packing it away, until the day my treatment ends. For you are no longer a person with specific traits, you're a patient who's expected to do whatever is asked of you.

The radiologist nicks my breast with a small scalpel, to aid with the insertion of the gun. He then proceeds to take four samples. The sound is reminiscent of my experience with a staple gun and a maple chair. I'm not surprised when he says: "It sure is hard." He's not telling me something I don't already know. Although I feel no pain, I do feel pressure, and the sound of the biopsy gun resonates as if striking something unyielding.

"I guess it's not a fatty tumour," I mutter — to no one in particular.

The radiologist remains quiet. He has said enough. Cancer is hard and, although the hardness can signify something other than cancer, it probably does not. He leaves the room without words or a second glance.

"It's all over," the female technician says as she flicks the lights on. She sees a trickle of blood run down my breast, and puts a Band-Aid on it. I nearly smile. It looks as if my breast has a little booboo. "Are you returning to work?" she asks.

"No, I'm going to a friend's house for coffee."

She touches my arm. "Good luck."

I now know I need it. I'm not one of the lucky five percent.

Judy brings out our favourite tarts. Strawberries, blueberries, and kiwis cover the custard in glazed glory. Her smile is satisfied, her eyes expectant. She thinks I'll announce we have cause for celebration. She pours two steaming mugs of coffee. The rich aroma tells me the coffee is from her secret cache — her Jamaican gold.

"I was right, wasn't I? It's a fatty tumour."

Her face is cheerful and eager. I don't want to pierce her self-made bubble of optimism with reality.

"They don't give you the results right away," I explain. "They have to biopsy them."

"Oh," she says, clearly disappointed. A second later, the wide smile is back. "Within the week, you'll find out that you don't have cancer."

I blow on my steaming coffee and nod.

We enjoy our visit and make small talk. She brings out empty packages, with illustrations. They fill the kitchen table.

"Look at the bulbs I planted," she says.

I see painted tulips, peony tulips, parrot tulips. A dizzying array of colours will herald her spring. I didn't buy bulbs this year. Hours pass. As I leave, she hands me reassurances, which are groundless. I step out the door and promise to call her when I get news.

Once home I start googling. I want to find out what sort of hard mass can reside in a breast and not be cancer. Until I hear the words, I'll continue to dream. I find a site on breast lumps.

A cyst feels smooth and squishy and there is some give to it, like a water balloon. It can move around and it changes size during your menstrual cycle. My lump is not soft and squishy, so cross out the cyst. Fibroadenomas, another kind of lump, are round, hard, and movable. I try to budge my lump and cannot decide if it moves. Fibroadenomas are located near the surface of the breast and you can easily feel them.

Mine seems deeper but I grip hope, until I read that it usually appears in teens and younger women. Fifty is not young. My personal summation amplifies when I read: Not common in postmenopausal women. I'm not post- but I am perimenopausal. All right then, next lump. Pseudolumps, much better. It sounds as if it is pretending to be a lump. Ha, ha, fooled you, you don't have cancer, you have a make believe bump, you knob. The good thing about pseudolumps is that they are benign. I especially like reading how they feel hard and do not change shape. They may or may not be moveable. My lump fits into that category, until I read it usually appears after breast surgery, or enhancement, or if a rib has shifted. I never had breast surgery and, although I would like to believe that a rib could shift without you knowing it, it sounds unlikely. The last lump on the list is breast cancer, which has an irregular shape, and a pebbly surface. It will be very hard and may not be movable. Since the tissue around it may move, it is difficult to know if it is moving. That doesn't help in the least. My lump is small; I can't tell if it is round or irregular in shape. It feels unmovable, but I'm not sure about that either.

Cancer always sounds substantial. No one has a little cancer. Instead, they have CANCER. In reality, the lumps and bumps are often small. It's the fear attached to them that makes them weighty.

The ultrasound results Fungus gave me described the lump as ill defined. Not the characterization one would use for a round mass. I want to ignore my rationale and wait for the results but I can't throw my worries away. I read people well. The radiologist's face showed embarrassment. He made a slip and knew it. The technician's touch held empathy. Not a good combination.

Stupid tests, stupid breasts.

*H*AVE YOU EVER gained unwanted weight? It's unsightly. You can feel it with every step you take, but you pretend the extra pounds aren't there. It's especially easy if it sits on your ass. Don't look back, and your smile can stay in place, even if your underwear doesn't. You often wake up and hope the weight magically disappeared, because you chose an apple for your snack yesterday, or you walked around the block with your dog last evening. I treat my cancer in the same manner.

When Dr. Fungus calls me a few days later, I know what I will hear but I pretend I don't.

"I'm sorry to tell you but you have invasive ductal carcinoma."

Okay, maybe I didn't know the exact words, but I did know she would tell me I have cancer.

The silent phone line sounds like bated breath. She expects a response. Perhaps a thud as my body falls to the floor, or a gasp, a litany of profanity or a simple "Oh My God". All she gets is: "I see."

"Do you have any questions?"

"Exactly what does that mean?"

"Ductal is the type of cells. Although all breast cancer starts in the lining of the milk ducts, some originate from the duct cells themselves, and others from the lubules that populate the ends of the ducts."

"So mine's ductal?"

"That's correct."

"Invasive, that's bad, right?"

"It sounds worse than it is. It simply means the cancer has grown outside of the duct."

"That would be the lump?"

"Exactly. Ductal cancer forms a hard lump because scar tissue around the cells causes a reaction. Seventy percent of breast cancer is invasive ductal. I've set up an appointment with Doctor Miller at the breast clinic. He's a plastic surgeon. You should be hearing from him in a few days. The clinic is very quick to call back."

Hadn't I heard that one before?

I didn't know what to say, other than goodbye. Only when the phone is in the cradle, do I wonder why I need a plastic surgeon. When it becomes clear, my chest recoils.

Fungus' words take away the straws I've been frantically clutching. My hand is as empty as the room I sit in. She didn't deliver her words in person. I'm alone. I'm officially sick. A phone call changes my life. Human contact is out of reach. Her job was made easier; mine, more difficult.

Did my ailment begin with the first cell's chaotic metamorphosis? The transformation started years past, without my awareness. As cells malign, I carry on as usual, oblivious to the havoc occurring under my very nose. The battle began without witness, without fanfare, without set boundaries, without allies. Cancer is underhanded in its plundering and it has an accomplice, for complacent ignorance buries the theft.

I'm outraged. How can my body do this to me?

Cancer's effectiveness lies in betrayal and deceit. Cancer is cowardly. It doesn't announce its presence. A sneaky thief, it slinks in darkness, free to steal what it pleases.

My brain is now aware of what has taken place. The doctor's words pierce my heart, and touch my soul, causing it to become frightened and discouraged. Is that the moment sickness takes hold?

I believe so, for poignant moments demand the partaking of the mind, body, and soul. Only then does the instance become real. A crime had been committed. My mind grasps the concept. Diverse emotions overrun my heart. Anger, fear, regrets, self-pity, they all impose themselves, as they fight to be at the front of the line.

Fungus called when everyone was at school or work. We began our conversation as the sun set. Although only minutes have passed, the house is now dark and ominous. I turn on the light.

I'm sick. I have cancer. I will fight it. I will win, for betrayal doesn't deserve to be victorious. Belatedly entering battle, I swear to be the victor.

I hurry to the computer. I search each term she used. I want to understand the enemy. For the hell of it, I do an online test that determines your risk of developing breast cancer. I ignore my diagnosis and fill in the questionnaire as if I hadn't heard Fungus' words. The results astound me. In the next five years, my risk of developing breast cancer is 1.1%. The average woman, the same age as me, has a score of 1.3%. My probability of not getting breast cancer in the next five years is a hefty 98.9%. My lifetime risk, using age ninety as my ceiling, is 9.9%. The average woman's score, to age ninety is 11.2%. My scores are better than the average woman's scores!

Just goes to show you that no one should feel as if they don't require a mammogram. Your risk may be low, but low doesn't mean it can't happen. Probability doesn't exclude possibility. Take the time to do the mammogram.

MY DIAGNOSIS CAME a day before my father-in-law's ninetieth birthday. I can be the ultimate party pooper.

Celebrate your ninetieth. My cancer doesn't change things.

Right. It will spoil everything. High spirits will shatter and re-arrange into guilt. My in-laws deserve their special day. My news can wait until Monday. My start day, the day I'll admit to everyone, including myself, I have cancer. Hearing the words aloud change my perceptions. I knew I had cancer from the beginning. Yet I continued to hope, until reality swept away the few crumbs I hoarded. Is optimism a gift or a form of stupidity?

My in-laws invite everyone to their house to share in Dino's birthday celebration, and his and Maria's sixtieth wedding anniversary. The two events are only weeks apart, so they're rolled into one. There will be more guests than they expect.

Their son, who lives in Toronto, is coming for the event with his family, as is Nadia, their oldest grandchild.

Luke has a birthday surprise for his father. He wrote to the Prime Minister explaining that his father is celebrating a milestone birthday. The Prime Minister sends a plaque congratulating Dino on living so long. The local television station announces the important birthday, the day before the celebration. When we arrive for the party, Dino tells Luke how he enjoyed the numerous calls he received. He heard from friends he hadn't heard from in years.

When Luke gives Dino the plaque, his father is thrilled. The Prime Minister sent something to him, imagine that. Dino stands tall and proud, but Luke towers over his father, even though he is only five-ten. Dino is a small man, only five foot five. Every one of his children is taller and sturdier, but none move as effortlessly or as quickly. Dino darts from person to person, showing off his accolade. Hard to believe that the little white haired man is ninety. His skin is unlined and his soul is youthful.

Twenty-five people sit around the dining room table. The table nearly overflows with the delectable food Maria prepared. Laughter fills the air, evoking memories of past pleasures. When the meal is over my son Zack asks: "What is the secret to such a long life, nonno?"

"Moderation," Dino says. "Eat and drink whatever you want, but never eat or drink too much." Good advice indeed, but he gives no mention to luck. If you live long it's because you lived well. If you die young, bad luck gets the blame.

"What about the secret to such a long and happy marriage?" Nadia asks.

"Never stop listening to each other," Maria says, and Dino smiles in agreement.

The couple sit close to one another. They stare into each other's eyes repeatedly, and often find reasons to touch one another. They're lucky to have their health, and each other. I feel a pang of envy, but I refuse to acknowledge it. The worst sickness comes from within. I must not allow envy to dampen my soul, for like moss, it can envelop everything, and envy's malevolence trumps cancer in its wickedness.

Their oldest son, Dominic, holds up his glass of wine. "To mom and pop, to their happiness, to their health." We all drink gladly.

ONDAY ARRIVES, THE word has to get out ... I'm a malignant tit. Damn it.

Luke cries when I tell him.

"I can't believe this is happening to you," he says, sobbing as he wraps me in his arms and holds tight.

"It seems surreal," I say. "When your trust in your own body shatters, it leaves you wobbly. I don't know what I can count on."

"You can count on me."

I hug him tighter. "I never doubted that."

"When did you find out?" he asks, realizing I must have known before that moment.

The hours I held the secret tight, feels deceitful. "I found out on Friday."

I feel his body stiffen. "And you didn't tell me."

I can see he's hurt. Sharing is the basis of our marriage. I took something, and made it my own. That's not how we do things.

"I didn't see the point of spoiling your family's celebration," I say.

Luke's mouth becomes tight. He appears nearly lipless. The line that cuts across his face tells me he's annoyed.

"This is much more important than a celebration."

"No, they're both equally important. If anything, rejoicing was exactly what I needed. Dousing their happiness wouldn't have helped me."

He remains quiet, but his annoyance dissipates with the onslaught of logic. "When are we going to tell the children?" he asks a moment later.

I've given a lot of thought to that question. In two days, I'll have my appointment with Doctor Miller.

"I would prefer to wait until we talk to the specialist. I don't feel I know enough to answer my own questions, let alone theirs."

"You're right, but I don't know if I can pretend nothing is going on."

Luke wears his heart on his sleeve. He's very transparent. I grab him by the shoulders.

"You have to be brave for me."

He nods, but I'm left wondering if I'm asking too much from him. When stoicism was handed out, not many Italians got in the line. I fear he'll do something obvious, like burst into tears and run from the room, but I needn't have worried. He finds strength, and the children never suspect a thing. Mind you, twenty-some-year-olds are not good at reading their parents. We're a dusty book they don't often look at.

On the day of my appointment with Doctor Miller, my son casually comes down the stairs. He's a university student and home all day. He sees Luke and me having coffee. He turns to his father and asks: "What are you doing home?"

Luke looks up from the newspaper.

"Your mother and I are deciding on what type of granite we want for the kitchen. We'll make our choice today."

Not a total lie. We're going to the doctor's first, and then the granite shop.

Luke feels bad for me. He wants me to have the granite countertops I always desired. I would prefer to stick with laminate and be cancer free, but I pretend to be excited about them. I know it's his way of doing something, in a situation where other than comfort me, he can't do very much at all.

Luke drives to the clinic. He holds my hand as we sit in the waiting room. I'm now one of the white women, with a terrified man sitting beside her. Damn it, I joined a club. I hate clubs.

The time of my scheduled appointment comes and goes. Finally, the doctor's nurse introduces herself and leads us into a conference room. We sit at a round table. Debra chats, and fills the table with pertinent pamphlets. She's a perky blonde with a warm disposition. She hands me a phone number. "Call me, if you have any questions." She smiles, and her blue eyes soften. "No question is irrelevant. You can call me about anything." She touches my hand. When I look into her face, I know she means what she says.

Pink walls surround us. They're reminiscent of my childhood bedroom. I'm usually derisive when it comes to anything ultra feminine. It stems from being dressed in pink for the first ten years of my life. *I get it, you had a girl.* Rather than being amused, I feel the surroundings are appropriate. Breast cancer is a woman's disease. Only two percent of breast cancer patients are males.

I glance at the wall clock. Debra notices.

"Doctor Miller is always late. He never rushes anyone, and will explain things as many times as he has to. He's very patient."

"There's a lot a person has to digest. I wouldn't want to be rushed when it's my turn to talk to him."

"Remember that when you're kept waiting. He's a great doctor but he falls behind quickly."

I value her answer. It makes sense and seems fair. Cancer puts people in an altered class. Time although valuable pales alongside the empathy cancer patients deserve. You can't only think of yourself. As you're growing impatient in a waiting room, someone in the next room could be receiving devastating news.

I get up and peer out the window. Arts and Craft homes line the street. I look at them, but I don't really see them. I think about my situation. A diagnosis of cancer is unforeseeable, unthinkable.

As if reading my thoughts, Debra says: "Cancer is an emotional disease. You fight the disease, but you also battle the feelings entrenched in the word itself. There's a saying around here. Cancer isn't a sentence. It's a word. And if you have to have cancer, breast cancer is the one to have. It's well funded. New treatments, and better diagnostics, are improving the survival rates with every passing year."

I turn from the window and wonder if the basic facts I've learned about breast cancer will enable me to follow Doctor Miller's summation of my circumstances.

The squeaking of the door tells me I will soon find out. Doctor Miller walks into the room. Everything about him is long and thin. He apologizes for his tardiness, introduces himself, and joins us at the table.

My experience with Doctor Fungus taught me not to automatically ascribe the trait of benevolence to a person, just because they're in the medical profession. Nonetheless, the tall thin man sitting beside me has kind eyes and a reassuring gentle manner. I especially like his tentative smile. He's a surgeon who saves lives daily, but he doesn't appear to ascribe importance to himself. I suspect he chose his specialty to help people, rather than to impress.

"I don't know how much you know about breast cancer," Doctor Miller says. "I'll give you a rudimentary summary of your situation." His voice matches his demeanour; it too is quiet and gentle.

"Rudimentary is good."

"The tumour isn't large, but it is substantial. Approximately two centimetres." He looks directly into my eyes. "You'll have surgery, because you do have a small cancerous lesion, and we always remove a cancerous mass. The good news is it doesn't appear to have spread to your lymph nodes. Nonetheless, I'll examine them during the surgery to make sure they haven't been affected. The big question today is what sort of surgery you want. We can perform a mastectomy or a lumpectomy."

When I found out my right breast was cancerous, I wanted the whole breast removed. Cancer be gone, was my emotional response. When fear eased up, I found information on the subject. Choices made in fear are often regretted. Visiting sites on the internet helped me become comfortable with my diagnosis. Cancer scares the sense out of you. Information and knowledge helps you look at it in the eye.

Most women have a mastectomy as their preliminary therapy for breast cancer. It relates to the fear factor. I asked myself a simple question: If I don't cut off the breast, will I lie awake every night and wonder if the cancer came back? I would not. I see my breast as containing a cancerous tumour. It is not cancerous. If the answer were yes, I would sever myself from my breast.

Surgeons once removed a large amount of skin when they did mastectomies. Reconstructions moved them into the practice of skin-sparing mastectomies. They now remove the breast and leave extra skin for reconstruction. Unless the woman concludes she won't have reconstruction. In that case, the surgeon won't leave you looking saggy. They'll trim the excess skin, and form a nice clean line across the chest. Removal of the breast doesn't trouble me as much as removal of the nipple. Maybe it's because I was never busty. However, I appreciate symmetry. Silly perhaps, but true.

I viewed pictures of women who had mastectomies (thank you) and read their personal accounts. They gave up their breast in exchange for feelings of safety and well-being. I understand their logic, but I can't see myself making the same choice. One woman diagnosed as stage 0 opted for a double mastectomy. The fear of reoccurrence outweighed her breasts. I thought it was overkill. She didn't. A personal choice.

The second option, the lumpectomy, starts with the removal of the lump, and the rim of normal tissue surrounding it. The goal is to ensure a clean margin. In other words, get the entire cancerous lesion. This is why Dr. Miller trained in oncoplastic surgery. His technique removes the tumour and allows the breast to be reconstructed cosmetically. (They don't add implants. More like putting Humpty Dumpty back together again). The two breasts should look alike, although depending on the size of the tumour, and the margin taken around it, one breast will be bigger than the other one. The drawback of a lumpectomy: radiation is mandatory. Radiation is not as debilitating as chemotherapy, but it's time consuming. You have to go to the hospital every day, Monday thru Friday, for three to five weeks.

I recite what I recently learned: "I've read that mastectomies and lumpectomies with radiation have the same success rate."

"That's correct. Years ago, we always performed a mastectomy when dealing with a cancerous growth. Since then we have learned that a lumpectomy with radiation is equally good at preventing a reoccurrence. Most surgeons prefer to conserve the breast whenever possible."

"I'm leaning towards a lumpectomy," I say. "I weighed my fear of reoccurrence against my desire to put this experience behind me. A lumpectomy will make cancer's signature less prominent, thereby making it easier to forget I was a victim of cancer."

Doctor Miller smiles, nods, and makes a notation in my chart.

"It's a personal choice unless the tumour is too large, especially in relation to a small breast. Or when there is more than one growth in the breast, and multiple lumpectomies are not possible. Mind you, chemotherapy prior to surgery can shrink the tumour, making a lumpectomy feasible."

My opinion matters to him. I respect him for that. I'm the one who will live with the outcome; it seems reasonable that I shouldn't have a passive role. I also value how Doctor Miller understands that laypersons have difficulty understanding his world.

"I don't see any problem with a lumpectomy," he says. "Given the size of the lump, and given that it doesn't appear to have spread, I think a lumpectomy is a good choice. I believe in conserving the breast whenever possible because, even though you can have reconstruction, it won't be your breast. There will be no sensation in the implant."

"But aren't you a hundred percent certain the cancer won't come back when you have a mastectomy?" Luke asks. Luke is a cautious person. If he had cancer, he would remove the whole part. He didn't try to dissuade me from my choice, but he made it clear if he were facing the same circumstances he would remove the breast.

"That's not necessarily so. Cancer can grow in the scar tissue of someone who has had their entire breast removed."

"What can you tell me about radiation?" I ask.

"When a lumpectomy is performed, we always cut a margin around the lump to ensure we have a clean margin. Nonetheless we can't be a hundred percent sure there are no cancer cells remaining. That is where radiation comes in. Radiation therapy uses energy from x-rays, gamma rays, electrons and other sources to destroy cancer cells. High doses ensure the destruction of cancer cells in the tumour bed. It damages the DNA in their genes, making it impossible for them to grow and divide. Unfortunately both cancer cells, which are growing in an uncontrolled way, and healthy cells are affected, but most healthy cells can repair themselves."

"What's the difference between radiation and chemotherapy?" Luke asks.

"There are a lot of differences. A major distinction is radiation destroys cancer cells in the breast, whereas chemotherapy targets cancer in any part of your body."

"So radiation is more localized?" Luke asks.

"Exactly It's also less toxic. It depends on the person, but radiation to the breast usually causes changes to the skin. Your breast may look sunburned or tanned. It may become red, irritated, or swollen. After a few weeks, your skin may become dry, or peel. It can even develop blisters. A treatment team will help you care for all of these problems.

Fatigue is also an issue. Your body is using a lot of energy to heal itself. You'll become tired. Daily trips to the hospital are also draining. The fatigue will cease gradually, after your treatment has ended."

Doctor Miller looks at us and awaits more questions. When none are forthcoming he says: "How do you typically do in surgery?"

"I usually do well."

"No problem with the anaesthetic?"

"No."

"Your lumpectomy should be day surgery, but I'll give you the option of spending the night. Besides the lumpectomy, I'll also be performing a sentinel node biopsy. This procedure removes one or more nodes, where the cancer is most likely to spread. I'll be making a second incision under your arm. You'll have your prognosis only after I've performed the surgery. The tumour and nodes must be removed and analyzed, before we understand what we're dealing with."

From the books I have read, I've learned Stage 1 is a T-1 tumour with no lymph nodes showing cancer. Stage 2 is either a small tumour with positive lymph nodes, or a tumour between 2 and 5 centimetres with negative lymph nodes. The latter example is often called 2A. Tumours between 2-5 centimetres, with positive lymph nodes, or tumours larger than 5 centimetres with negative lymph nodes, are also stage two but they are judged stage 2B. Stage 3 is a large tumour with positive lymph nodes, or a tumour with grave signs. Grave signs are swollen lymph nodes, large tumours, ulceration and swollen skin (looks dimpled like an orange). A Stage 4 tumour has spread to other parts of the body.

Doctor Miller classes my tumour as a Stage 2A.

"Before surgery you'll meet the anaesthesiologist. You'll also have blood work, and your heart will be checked. I'll schedule you for a MRI. I like to have a clear picture of what I'll find, before I go in, and the MRI is the most sensitive of tests. If you don't mind, I would like to go next door and perform an examination."

Doctor Miller checks my breast, collarbone area, and armpit. Oncologists who specialize in breast cancer spend a lot of time prodding armpits. I don't want to sweat, so buckets of perspiration drip from my pores. Whenever you exude something obnoxious, you're told it's good for you. I retch after surgery and nurses often nod and say: "It's a good thing. Your body is ridding itself of the medications. Consider it a cleansing process." Rather difficult to feel clean when puke clings to your hair in foul smelling blobs.

Sweat releases toxins. I sit on the table and feel like a nuclear waste plant. Doctor Miller pretends not to notice. The gentle air that surrounds him is genuine. I'm in good hands. He's as kind and caring as his eyes claim him to be.

Fungus was a bad start but I won't allow her to blemish the kind, warm-hearted doctors I meet.

$\mathcal{A}$FTER DOCTOR MILLER answers all our questions, Debra wants to introduce us to the social worker, Linda. Her specialty is helping women cope with breast cancer. I don't want to meet the woman. However, I don't want to appear cantankerous either. Who wants to be cancerous and cantankerous?

I try my best to assure Debra I don't need a social worker. "I can talk to my loving family and many friends."

She counters with: "It helps to meet women facing the same situation."

What can I say? Unable to counter her counter with a counter, I nod and find myself sitting across from Linda.

I'm not emotional. Tears, wailing—what's the point? It won't accomplish anything. I like to be polite. I like to pretend I have a nice disposition. I appear to be an extrovert, whereas I'm an introvert with social skills. Eysenck should have had two groups for introverts; some of us have social skills, but prefer not to use them. I favour not surrounding myself with people. If pressed for a definitive answer to: Do you like people?, I would have to qualify: Which people?

Luke and I smile at Linda. She begins to speak. Yada, yada ... She talks about how my diagnosis makes me feel and I half listen. She never experienced breast cancer yet books told her how I should feel. I don't discount her education. I'm sure she has helped countless women. But a book is different from the actual experience.

My education began early in life. At eleven, life taught me how you can't take anything for granted. A sunny warm July day, a hurried kiss on the cheek—that's my last memory of my father. I went to the theatre with my mother. We returned to find my daddy dead from a heart attack. The doctor had just given him a clean bill of health. Fool me once ...

Linda talks about how I'll break the news to my children.

"They are actually young adults," I say.

"What about your parents?"

Within five minutes, Linda hands me a Kleenex. She found my Achilles heel and is presently assuring me loved ones can cope with the news that yes

~ *your wife has cancer*
~ *your daughter has cancer*
~ *your mother has cancer*
~ *your best friend has cancer*

Hurting the ones I love is worse than the diagnosis of cancer. I have to spread its filthy tentacles and I despise being in its thrall. I cry. The tears are not born of sadness but out of frustration and anger.

When I was a teenager, I would talk to a girl after school, once the buses left the yard, and no one was around. We were unlikely friends but camaraderie developed nonetheless. After weeks of sharing secrets, laughing, complaining, and getting to know each other well, Karen stunned me when she said she didn't want to be my friend anymore.

"Why not?" I ask. I find her witty and forthright. I enjoy our conversations and assume she does too.

"Being my friend is dangerous," she says.

"Dangerous, what do you mean?"

"Everyone knows I'm the school slut. If they see us hanging out together, they'll think the same of you."

Her reputation is well known. She is promiscuous but she is also astute, funny, and sensitive.

"I don't care what people think. You're a nice person. I like talking to you. We always have a good time together. Why let anyone ruin it?"

"I like you too. That's why I'm never talking to you again."

"But ..."

Her pretty face turns mean.

"No buts. You're naive. Do you want my reputation?"

"It's not something you can catch," I say. "You're more than that, and if people are too stupid to see it, that's their problem."

Her face softens. She once again looks like my friend. "Actually it will be your problem."

I square my shoulders and jut my chin. "If I'm not worried about it why should you be?"

"It's like I said, I like you. You're a sweet girl."

She walks away. She doesn't turn around when I call her name. She's true to her word. Karen never speaks to me again. She tossed our friendship away, as if it were dirt. I never forgive her.

My new friend is cancer. Cancer won't walk away. It will define me. I am malignant. Being a slut, or being cancerous, is not something people can overlook. Malignancy will label me. It will change how people think of me. No one can pull me away from its grasp.

My cancer will also affect those around me. I'm sorry about that, but I'm powerless.

"It's not your fault you have cancer," Linda says. "Your loved ones can gather strength and they will be happy to help you. Make them feel useful. Give them something constructive to focus on."

I don't blame myself. I'm a victim. The trap I'm in is not of my doing. My life spins out of control, as cancer pushes me aside, and takes front and centre stage. Cancer is grave. Cancer demands honesty. I must introduce it to everyone in my life. To disregard its appearance is unforgiveable. I can spare no one. I will follow Linda's advice and give each of them a job to do. Provide the illusion that they can help me. I resent the hurt I'll cause. I resent my role of fear monger. I resent being sick. I resent being ... weak. Cancer tells me how to live my life. Who gives it the right? My fucked up body that doesn't know how to behave itself, that's who. I'm not scared. I'm too busy being angry.

Luke and I decide to tell the children after dinner. The following day I'll tell my mother.

We leave Linda's office, our hands full of books, and pamphlets and phone numbers, contacts for gym memberships, women's support groups, libraries, help lines, cancer forums, hook-up with survivors ...

NIGHTMARES CIRCLE THE world. Common premises land and elicit identical fears in everyone, everywhere. Regardless of age, our slumber often transports us back to school where a test educes a pounding heart.

Your glance is stupid, as you stare at the handout. The subject matter is unfamiliar. Dread fills you until you feel nothing else. You cannot pass this test. The environment is alien. The teacher is a stranger. Students talk among themselves, ignoring you, making you feel invisible and impotent. Importance thickens the air. It hovers over you; its largeness makes you feel insignificant. Instincts kick in. Something monumental is about to take place. Something you are not prepared for.

Agitated, scared, and disoriented, you tell yourself: it can't be happening. If you knew you were to be tested, you would have prepared.

Telling the people I love I have cancer transports me into that nightmare. My eyes are open, yet I'm taken unaware. I feel ill equipped. Reality seems surreal. Nothing I have ever experienced prepares me emotionally for the task.

I read everything I can about breast cancer. I want answers to their questions. I want to pull powerlessness from them. I feel my responses will in part determine how they feel. I want to be reassuring. I want my answers to be optimistic. My words will hit their heart first, and optimism spears hope. Concrete facts must be the basis of my words. The brain resumes working, after the initial shock.

We sit in the family room. My children are by my side. I jump right in.

"I've just found out I have breast cancer."

I'm a charging bull. I no longer try to change my bluntness. It's how I deal with life. But what am I suppose to do ... initiate a guessing game?

Disbelief coats their faces. They hope they've misunderstood.

Got Brisk in the can sir? No, no, no, you heard right. I have breast cancer.

My son Zack speaks first: "When did you find out?"

I tell him.

"Why didn't you say anything?" my daughter asks. Her voice sounds accusatory. Why did I keep such a secret?

"I didn't want to scare you until I knew it was real."

Anger flashes. Have I made a mistake?

"Oh my God," Madison mutters. Fear displaces anger. Difficult to stay mad at a cancer victim. I'm sure there's a passage on it in a book of etiquette.

"I had hoped we wouldn't have this talk," I say. "I wanted to have the one where I was scared for nothing."

"I don't believe this," Zack says, as he folds his muscular arms. He sounds angry. He's a young man at the peak of his physical power. He stands six foot one and can bench press large weights. Helplessness was once a stranger.

"What's the prognosis?" Madison asks. Madison takes after my side of the family. She has childish features, and looks much younger than she is. I remind myself that I'm talking to a young woman, not a high-school student.

"It's very good. They're going to cut out the lump and then I'll have radiation."

"Why did this happen to you?" I strain to hear her words. I understand her sentiment. No one wants to recognize the face of a cancer victim, even when it is your own face staring back at you.

"I don't know," I answer. "If you calculate the risks, I actually scored lower than the average woman. No one in my immediate family had breast cancer; I had my children young in life, my menstrual cycle started at twelve. I exercise, am not overweight, and don't drink. Sometimes things just happen." I want to add that I have an asshole breast. It played dead most of its life. Only woke up to grow a tumour. It's too trite. How many underachievers turn bad? It remains unsaid.

Zack keeps asking questions. He nods and says: "I see," after each response. His face is devoid of emotion. I know what he's doing. I do it too. I don't sob, cry, or break down. Instead, I become analytical. Migraines, stomach problems, and the flu usually trail my stoic demeanour. Take it from a rock; we crumble from the inside out. I'll have to talk to Zack. I hope he'll reach out to me, or someone else.

Saying very little, Madison listens intently. Interlopers lose authority with knowledge.

I have cancer. We will get through it. Cancer will not terrorize us. I decide that from the very beginning. Am I arrogant? Maybe, but that's what I want to believe. I cannot be powerless. I will not be powerless, regardless of the strength of my opponent.

I'm not worried about Madison. She's a problem solver. She reaches out to others when she is scared or hurt. Once the shock wears off, she'll devise a plan of action. When she needs to talk, she will, but probably not to me.

Cancer creates a paradox. When it enters the picture, it alters the image by asserting itself over its victim, changing everyone's perception of the individual. It strips you of your individuality. You become cancer. Your loved ones want you back. They hold tight in a desperate attempt to free you from its grip. They try to drive the cancer away, by sharing strength, as they will you to get better.

However, when they're weak, they move away. They shield you from their negative energy. Fearful it will empower the cancer. The dance step is basic. Feeling optimistic, take a step forward, for good feelings shrink cancer. If you feel pessimistic, take a step back, because bad feelings are cancer's nourishment. Actions rather words reveal the code.

It will take the passing of months before my daughter admits, the night I revealed my cancer, she hid in the pantry to cry, without letting a tear fall, or a sound escape.

Shielding affirms itself upon the arrival of cancer. My children now see me as weak. They become strong. I want to protect them. They're determined to protect me. They'll hold me tight, or release me, as cancer spins our world up, down and all around.

When I look back, I wonder if we were brave or stunned. Do you digest bad news in tiny bites? Does acceptance only take place when you swallow the last mouthful?

Luke joins us. Later he admits to being hurt because I didn't include him in breaking the news. I don't know why I chose to tell my children without the presence of their father. I think it's because I wanted to tell them in my own way, because it's my cancer. It takes me awhile to realize cancer is something you share. We hug one another. Our solidarity strengthens us. The illusion of others helping me is turning out not to be an illusion at all. Cancer forces me to realize we all need others, regardless of how independent we think we are.

My mother is the one I dread telling the most. Not because she's older, weaker, or the one I love the most. It's because she lives alone.

Widowed at forty-two, rather than accept assistance, Mom found a low paying job and worked fifty-hour weeks to put food on the table, and keep a roof over our heads. I don't doubt her strength but I know her weakness: me, her only child, who took twelve years of marriage to conceive. You don't touch my mother's baby.

I invite her for lunch. Once we're having our coffees, I tell her my news. I can read the emotions she feels, as her brain processes my words. Shock, fear, sorrow, and finally resolution, flash in her black eyes. Yet she will not scare me. The first words out of her mouth are: How can I help you?

I grab her hand and squeeze. "I don't know but we'll find out."

My mother looks older after our talk. She's eighty-one but normally looks seventy. Her youthful freckled face helps her retain the vestiges of youth. She has strong cheekbones and an animated face. Presently she looks drawn.

When Madison comes home from work, we discuss mundane things. My mother, like me, doesn't like to stay anywhere very long. She begins to fidget. I know she wants to go home and deal with the news in seclusion. She wants to shed tears, but she won't allow me to see a demonstration of her pain and fears. My mother stands five feet tall. Arthritis riddles her body. Look into her black eyes and you do not see a small, weak woman. My mother is large in spirit, and tough in character.

"Madison, would you mind driving Grandma home?"

"Sure thing," she says. Lately my children do everything I request of them. Mothers around the world wonder how to get their children to obey without nagging. The answer is simple: get cancer. Children might be lazy and disobedient but they love you. Illness shows them and you how much. I rather be cancer free and nag everyone to death. There are worse things than disobedience and laziness.

When I hear the car door shut and the engine start, I hurry to the computer. I email my mother's sister. I tell her about my breast cancer. I ask her to call my mother, later that night, and to pretend not to know anything. I do it because I feel my mother needs to talk to someone about her fears. My mother and I share a very close relationship. But the person she needs is not me. I'm one of the unwell. I'm now part of a distinct society.

Months later Madison tells me that, as soon as they round the corner, my mother insists she stop the car. Mom's arthritic body battles knee-deep snow. She makes her way to the garbage can, at the entrance of the park. She throws up violently and stumbles back to the car.

"If you felt sick, why didn't you use our bathroom?" Madison asks.

"Don't tell your mother I threw up."

What is wrong with my family? When upset we don't cry, we puke. Like really, you will never see that reaction in the movies. Can you imagine *Gone With the Wind* if Scarlett was a family member of mine?

"Sue, I'm sorry for everything. I should have been a better sister," Scarlett sobbed after a long while in silence. She then grabbed a bucket and retched violently. Afternoon tea and scones lined the bucket in a congealed rank mess. Vomit flew across the room in an unsightly arc.

Suellen frowned and shook her head. The smell caused her to cough. In between coughs, she quietly said: "Don't worry anymore. What's done is done. That's the past, and it's gone now. What's important is ..." Her strength took that precise moment to fail her. Sheer determination forced the words to flow from her mouth. "What's important is removing that bucket from the room. It's making my stomach churn." She grimaced. Scarlett leaned over her and kissed her gently on the cheek. Suellen could smell her fetid breath and feared she too would vomit. As if dying was not bad enough.

Suellen looks into her sister's eyes. "You are so beautiful. Stay beautiful. Learn to be happy. Let the past go dear. All the ugliness, it's gone now. Time for something new. Tell Rhett how much you love him and start new ... And most importantly of all, brush your teeth."

Scarlett's tears overflowed. If only she could tell Rhett. She felt Suellen's hand go limp in hers as her eyes closed for the last time. She was gone.

Death did not bring serenity to her sister's face. Suellen looked repulsed. Death must be repugnant, Scarlett decides. Scarlett staggered away from her dead sister.

Mammy woke up to gurgling sounds of Scarlett's retching. She moved across the room to comfort her Scarlett and take her away from the sight in front of her, to her room, where she needed to rest up a bit but Mammy slipped on the puke that made walking treacherous. Mammy crawled away. She had wanted to protect Scarlett, but at the moment thought: My dear I don't give a damn. I ain't changing that bed or mopping that floor.

It is abundantly clear why there is not one thespian in our family tree.

$\mathcal{N}$OW THAT THE nuclear family knows I have cancer, I have to tell friends and the rest of the relatives. I don't have to tell my cousin Carole, whom I think of as a sister, because her mother called her right after she read my e-mail.

Carole immediately calls me. "Whenever you need something, whenever you have to talk, cry, shout or complain, think of me. I want to be there for you because I love you. I'm your big sister so there is nothing you can ask of me that I wouldn't give."

I can't say anything because, other than anger, I have difficulty expressing my emotions. She manages to elicit a promise to keep her abreast of the situation.

Kindness makes me clam up. Intense emotions cause me to shrink. Deep down, I know I fear them. I also know why. I lost too many loved ones when I was a child. Pretty much broken, as soon as I was taken out of the box. I'm terrified to love because I can't bear the pain of parting. I can appear cold, whereas in reality I'm easily hurt. No one knows this because I lick my wounds in secrecy and never allow tears to fall.

When I tell my best friend Judy my news, she seemingly takes it well. "You will get through this. You're strong and the advancements in breast cancer allow women to beat it. It's not what it once was. There are more survivors with every passing year."

She goes on to tell me about her friend who had breast cancer and survived. I never suspect her brave face hides fears. Months later her daughter tells me how my illness was not mine alone. While I was undergoing tests and treatments, Judy battled insomnia and migraines. She was literally sick with worry. Only when I was on the road to wellness did she find her way to better health. Judy joined me on my journey and I never knew it. I guess we're two broken toys.

My mother in law cries when my husband tells her the news. In the past, she often had the knack of saying all the wrong things to me.

On this occasion, she makes up for it. "Be strong; believe the outcome will be good. Don't scare yourself, empower yourself instead. You can beat this. I will pray for you."

When elderly Italian women promise to pray, they ain't kidding. Her rosary beads appear smaller by the time I have a clean bill of health.

Sometimes friends and relatives run away from sick individuals. I'm lucky. No one of consequence falls in this group. But some have difficulty expressing themselves. A close friend admits to being shocked and unable to find words. Far from eloquent, she stumbles upon hearing the news. Nonetheless, she manages to convey that she's my friend and always will be. Some never bring up the topic of cancer but, whenever something needs doing, they are there.

16

*H*AVE YOU NOTICED that, whenever something happens to you, you begin to see others in the same situation? You break your arm. Everyone around you seems to be wearing a cast. You become pregnant. Everyone is in maternity clothing.

I never knew anyone who had breast cancer. Suddenly I see them everywhere. I'm not talking about the women I meet at the breast clinic. I'm talking about the general population.

I just receive my diagnosis, and Jackie, a close friend of Madison, confides: "We just found out my mother has breast cancer."

Madison immediately says: "My mother has breast cancer too."

The news astounds them both. Madison gets queasy when she thinks of a knife cutting through skin.

"I don't know when my mom is having surgery," Jackie says. "They found three tumours. She has to do chemo first."

Madison doesn't know what to say. I have only one tumour. It's small. She now understands how cutting something out can be a good thing.

The girls talk. Jackie's mother is having difficulty coping, physically and emotionally, with the disease. Madison doesn't tell Jackie how well I'm doing.

Friends and family congratulate me for my courage.

I don't deserve it. What Jackie's mother is going through is different from my situation. She's not getting a lump removed; she's fighting for her life. She faces months of chemo, and her future is uncertain. Her lymph nodes are involved. A year ago, a mammogram shows nothing. Twelve months later, she has three tumours in one breast. Her tumours are much more aggressive than Spike. They're Rottweilers. My snarly little terrier is only snapping at my heels.

There's talk of a double mastectomy. She loses her hair; she loses her appetite; she loses her vitality; and finally, she loses her faith. Who can blame her when she's so weak she can barely get out of bed some days?

Cancer victims stand under the same umbrella, but the raindrops that fall around us are unique. Some fall straight down, barely touching us. Others seep under the umbrella and coat us with a fine mist. Rain can also pelt with an intensity that collapses umbrellas, leaving you numb and chilled. Unless you're standing under the umbrella, you can't understand the weight of the bombardment and the touch of the raindrops.

17

ANCER CHANGES PEOPLE and not just the person diagnosed with the disease. My mother, a poster girl for introverts, is suddenly talking to all the women in her building.

Her condominium is not a senior home, but many seniors live there. They all know I have breast cancer. Mother's behaviour stuns me. After the initial shock, I'm pleased. In her circle of friends, three have beaten breast cancer. Not to mention those with sisters who have also beaten the disease.

Her friends share their experiences with her. Scars are bared. They speak the same language as my mother. Clearer understanding results from the simple words stripped of medical jargon. One woman beat the disease twenty-five years ago. Another's battle took place five years ago. Each describes how they moved on. There is life after cancer!

"Everything will turn out just fine," my mother says, as she pats my arm. A steely look in her eyes makes them gleam. "You will win this battle." Those wonderful women took her fear and replaced it with hope and determination. I am awed and grateful.

Mom then goes on to explain: "The surgery isn't that bad. You'll heal quickly but you have to do the exercises or your arm will swell. You're young so you'll beat it."

I'm glad she reached out to her friends, but I must say I'm bowled over when the superintendent of her building wishes me luck on my MRI.

How many people are sharing my cancer with me?

My aunt has her congregation praying for me every Friday. One of the women makes me a quilt of soft cotton materials. Each square has pink in it. It's a quilt designed by a woman for a woman. Everyone says women can be catty and mean to one another, which is true. However, when you find yourself in need, a woman's arms reach out promptly and surely.

One Saturday afternoon Luke and I visit my aunt. The three of us pass the day shopping at small boutiques. People on the street smile and wave at us; some ask about my treatment. They're strangers, but they take a moment to wish me luck, or recount a story of a cancer survivor. I've heard many say the world is uncaring. It can be. Yet it is also loving and nurturing. I don't disregard the good, and focus on the bad.

I prefer to focus on the good. I do things to make me happy, solely because it makes me happy. I decorate dinner tables with fancy napkins, candles, and interesting china. Some see it as superficial and a waste of time. The food tastes the same, they remark. I don't see my love for beauty as shallow. The fancy trappings cover an interest I have in those around me. Candles, china, and napkins are not important. Creating, appreciating and wanting to bring a smile to another's face is the crux. What is life if daily acts are immaterial? Small acts are life.

Flowers cheer me up. In the wake of their design, my troubles seem inconsequential. Prior to surgery, I need to see flowers. I don't intend to buy any. I want to smile at old friends, and perhaps see some new faces. The nursery I frequent has an older Pakistani man who appears to live at the store. Whenever I visit, he's there.

I open the door to the nursery and I see Sammy in a far corner. He sees me, runs over, and wraps his arms around me. We're usually friendly with one another, but not that friendly.

"I'm so sorry to hear about your illness," he says. I have no idea how he found out.

"Thank you for your concern."

He looks at me and smiles widely. "Muslims pray a lot," he informs me. "We pray many times a day."

I return the smile and look down at him. He's a short, thin man.

"We will pray for you. I will get everyone at the Mosque to pray for you. You will get better."

"Thank you," I say automatically.

He grabs my hand. I feel the strength behind his scrawny frame.

"No, we will pray for you and you will get better."

His voice has risen. Conviction strengthens his words. He looks at me in a way that dares me to disagree. I nod in acquiesce. I feel better and I've yet to look at their stock. Flowers come in all shapes.

That night as I'm falling asleep, I envision the Catholics, Anglicans, and Muslims praying for me. The picture feels reassuring and makes me smile.

18

*J*HE WAIT TIME for an MRI can be unbelievably long, unless you have cancer and/or are willing to go in at an odd time. Mine is scheduled a week after Doctor Miller's appointment. I have to arrive by 8:50 p.m.

Madison insists on coming with me. "You can drive on the way there, but after the procedure, I'll drive you home."

As of late, she has become protective of me. My child is babying me, and her fretting feels ill fitting. Nonetheless, I'm happy to have company as we drive down the dark roads.

When we arrive, the clerk hands me forms and a clipboard. "Fill them out and return them to me," he says as he finds my name on the schedule. He points to the waiting room.

The forms include an illustration of two breasts. They ask you to indicate the location of your tumour. Madison laughs when I draw a circle and add pointy ears and a mean mouth to my cancer.

Cans rattle and thump, as people feed dollars to the soda machine in the hallway.

"I'm thirsty," Madison says as she hunts for a dollar in her disorganized purse.

I find a dollar and hand it to her.

She ambles over to the dispenser. Madison is frequently slow moving. I watch her and try to observe her with the eyes of a stranger. She's an attractive young woman, with long brown wavy hair, a petite frame, and an easy smile. The drink falls, and she grabs it and pulls its tab. Madison quaffs most of the orange soda in her first gulp. The orange liquid outlines her lips with its intense colour. She walks back and sits beside me. I fight the urge to hug my baby girl, and wipe her mouth.

As I finish filling out the form, a nurse wearing eggplant scrubs with black side panels enters the waiting room. "Nancy Burns," she calls out. I stand up, and she sees the forms in my hands. "I'll take those."

Her badge reads Stephanie.

I follow her to the changing room, adjacent to the MRI machines. I steal a glance, as I leave Madison behind. Bye bye, baby girl. Wipe your mouth yourself. I want to see you as a woman. I need to see you as grown up.

We arrive at the lockers. Stephanie hands me two gowns. "One ties in the back, the other in the front. You can retain your underwear, but the jeans have to go. You can put your belongings in a locker."

My mouth falls open and I turn away from her. Shit ... I assumed I would keep my jeans. A rather stupid assumption considering they have a zipper and a metal button. MRI, the M stands for *Magnetic*. Hello. Why did I make such an assumption? I guess I was too lazy to think. I'll pay for my mistake. I didn't shave my legs. The hairs dart outwards like spines on a cactus. To make matters worse, I'm wearing short dorky stockings. Damn, if only I'd worn high stockings. My mistake is blatant for everyone to see. I wear Spongebob socks, have cancer, and hairy legs.

Women sit in a row. Each wears gowns identical to mine. Lockers hold our personal belongings. We no longer wear the clothing others wear. Inhibitions that restrain fall from us, to land on the cold tiles beneath our feet. The person we are stands outside the door. A transformation begins once you walk through these doors.

The gown transcends age, race, and socioeconomic class. Such pithy variables recede in the wake of fear. Sit beside someone. It takes but a second to learn how they ended up in such a place. You discover their ailment, the degree of suffering they're afflicted with, and when the horror began, before the clock's small hand can move to the next hour.

Personas rest in a corner. Tossed aside and ignored. No subject is taboo. You hear about relationships with mates, siblings, children, and parents. Only one question remains unanswered: *Who are you?*

I was unaware of the omission until I began telling stories about the women I met.

Madison listens to my account. She interrupts my tale. "Mom you shouldn't refer to her as brain tumour. She has a name."

My head tilts as I think back on my conversation with brain tumour. I know there's a good chance she'll die. Pain batters her head and makes her scream. Her husband often cries and holds her tight as they try to sleep. I think back on all the conversations I've had. I know so much about the lives of strangers. I know their habits, loves, hates, fears. But names? I don't have any of those.

People share their disease but keep their healthy self at bay. We turn into doppelgangers — healthy and sick versions of ourselves. Weakened by illness, our doppelganger reaches out for help, as our healthy self closes its eyes, intent on remaining in the background, intent on remaining anonymous, intent on remaining untouched, free of the stain of sickness.

I sit beside an eighty-some-year-old woman. She is small and thin and her white hair looks professionally styled. Her name is ductal cancer. Her christening was in 1970.

"They only took out the tumour," she explains.

"No margin, no radiation?"

"No, they cut it out. I went home, had a smoke, and called it a day. They wanted me to cut off the whole breast, but I refused. I'm glad I did. That breast never got into trouble again. This time it's the other side."

It took forty years for the cancer to find her again. However, this time she's older and wiser and her cancer is duct cancer in situ. In other words, stage 0. It's just beginning while her lifespan is winding down.

"The doctor wants to keep an eye on it. It may not even develop into cancer." She suddenly sighs. "My husband came with me. I hope he's not too worried. He has a heart condition."

I think back of the people in the waiting room. "Is he wearing a plaid cap?" I ask.

"Yes."

"He asked the receptionist to change the television channel to the hockey game. He was cheering for Ottawa." My answer makes her smile.

"He loves hockey. Drives me crazy," she says with a roll of her eyes. "Hockey is all he thinks about." She pretends to be annoyed but I suspect the calmness has to do with his mind being on the game, not her.

This is where the guilt comes in. When the social worker told me not to feel guilty about having cancer, I thought: Don't be stupid, I don't. It's not as if I went shopping and said: *"Hey, can you give me something that will scare the shit out of my family?"*

"Sure thing, here's some breast cancer. That should do the trick."

"That's perfect, they deserve a good jolt."

I don't feel guilty about having the disease. I don't see it as my fault. Illness is not a choice.

Culpability arrives when the people who love you pay for that love with sorrow, fear, and anger. Love is something you share. It's a positive emotion, until sickness rears its head, and it transforms into a punishment. Your pain becomes their pain. Love secures your destiny with theirs. It makes you feel responsible.

We begin talking about her first bout with cancer. The story ends suddenly when a technician leads us to another room. The room houses chairs, tables, and an array of needles. I sit in a chair that resembles a lazy boy.

"This won't hurt," the technician says, as she inserts a needle into my arm. Attached to it is tubing. She's hooking me up so that, when I'm in the MRI, they'll be able to inject dye into my veins. The cancer will expose itself.

Only minutes pass before a door opens and the technician stands beside me and leads me through. The machine takes centre stage. It looks like a mouth with its tongue sticking out. I feel curiosity, not fear.

The technician is thirtyish, capable, but personable. She stands beside the tongue. "Take off your gowns, and lie down on your stomach."

I remove the gowns and hop onto the tongue.

"Put your arms over your head."

My breasts hang down into cup holders. They fit snugly. Do large breasted women overfill the cups? If they do, what happens? Perhaps the technician gives them the once over and guesses the appropriate vessel needed to house their breasts.

You look like a bucket to me. And you over there, a thimble will suffice.

Once I'm in place, a button is positioned near my right hand.

"If you feel anxious, press it, but remember if you do, the test will stop and we'll have to begin all over again." I nod. It's not hard to see that pressing the button will make things worse. Rather anxiety-producing instructions to give someone you want to remain calm. It doesn't matter to me. I won't press the button. Small spaces don't scare me. Encircling me tightly makes me feel secure.

"It'll be loud," the technician warns as she hands me a set of headphones. Like the johnnies, they must be one size fits all. They're too big and make me feel child-like. A button is pushed and I begin my journey into the machine. It's very bright inside and I know when they inject the dye into my veins because a stream of warmth spreads through me that is oddly comforting. The heat abates the constant ache I feel since having my breast biopsy. I've never told anyone about the pain but, when no one is home, I use a heating pad to obtain relief.

Sheltered, wrapped in warmth, I'm alone, but only for a second. My imagination joins me and suddenly I'm superwoman, flying through the air. Disconnected, I soar through the white light that remains, even though my eyes are closed. I'm temporarily happy and safe. It is only when the sounds stop that I pitch back to earth and land with a thud. I'm not a superhero. I'm a woman preparing for surgery.

"You'll be notified of the time for your ultrasound," the technician tells me as she leads me to the locker room. "It is standard procedure."

I'd never heard of having another ultrasound prior to taking the MRI. Instead of feeling like Superwoman, my spidey senses tingle, alerting me of personal danger. While the machine wrapped me in its warmth, it uncovered something. What, I do not know.

Cancer makes you paranoid but being paranoid is not equivalent to being wrong. The MRI was supposed to be the last test before surgery. Something has changed. The technician's face reveals nothing. She's not an easy read. Prior to the test, she appeared much more open. She's locking something up. Bad news?

I get dressed and return to the waiting room. Madison asks for the keys. I refuse to hand them over.

"I'm fine. I want to drive us home."

A hurt look flashes in her eyes, but she smiles nonetheless. I know I should let her drive. I can't. I need to be in control. I have to have power over something because I feel powerless and afraid. What did the machine learn? Why was I not privy to the information? Blunt and impatient, I hate beating around the bush. Protocol stopped the technician from telling me what they uncovered. It doesn't lessen my annoyance because protocol doesn't just beat around the bush. It escorts you through the whole garden, up the road, and around the town. Protocol, protocol ... What a pain in the ass.

I WAIT FOR the call about scheduling another ultrasound. It never comes. I assume the technician made a mistake.

I hear nothing about the results of the MRI. Silence reassures me. I was mistrustful without reason. There was nothing to see, talk about, or test. Silly, silly me.

Just when you think it's safe to go back in the water ...

I receive the call five days before my scheduled surgery. Three weeks after my MRI. I recognize my surgeon's voice. I glance to the time. Eight at night.

"The results of your MRI were sent to your general practitioner (Fungus). I never received them. Until now."

I remain silent. I don't like how this is unfolding. Surgeons do not call you on a Sunday evening.

"There appears to be a second tumour," Doctor Miller informs me. "It's at the ten o'clock position. We have to discuss how to proceed and, as much as I despise having this conversation on the phone, time restraints leave me no other choice. I'm leaving the country tomorrow morning and arriving back just in time for your scheduled surgery."

He keeps apologizing about the mix-up. His response is so different from my family doctor.

"What are my choices?"

"We can proceed with your scheduled surgery, and then look into the MRI results after the surgery."

"That could mean two surgeries, if the second lump proves to be cancerous."

"Yes, but we have no way of knowing if it is until we do a biopsy."

"I have one cancerous lump, so isn't it likely that the second one is also cancerous?" I'm beginning to think my breast isn't meant to be saved. *Bye, bye boobie, goodbye. Bye, bye boobie, don't cry.* The musical playing in my head is not entertaining in the least. I silence the orchestra.

"It's not necessarily malignant. It might be benign, or as I told you before, the MRI is too sensitive. The second mass could be a false positive."

A fake conclusive? Categorically bogus? Umm ... Something to ponder. Or not? *Should I try to save my breast? As of late, it has been a royal pain in the ass.*

"What's my other option?" I ask. I already know the answer and hold my breath.

"You could have a mastectomy."

Maybe I should. Many women have mastectomies. If it meant saving my life, I would not hesitate. But, is the second mass cancerous? Doctor Miller doesn't assume it is. What do we know about this second mass? We have suspicions, but nothing concrete. Are the results positively false? Or are they depressingly true?

It's consorting with a known malignancy, so in all probability it too is malignant. Is that the best logic? Maybe, but I can't give up my breast just yet. I think of Karen and how hasty generalizations cause unnecessary losses.

It's a difficult boob, but it's mine. If I have a mastectomy and the MRI findings turn out to be nothing, I'll regret my hurried decision.

"If I wait, will I be putting my life in jeopardy?"

"Cancer doesn't grow so quickly that a few weeks will make a difference. If you decide to give up your surgical slot, I'll immediately book another ultrasound and another MRI with a biopsy."

"Let's do that," I whisper.

Great, the nightmare will continue.

"Fine, someone will call you tomorrow and I'll try to get things to move as quickly as I can. I'm so sorry, but I think you're right in waiting. You want to make an informed decision. Without further testing we don't know your situation."

My MRI didn't make things clearer. It muddied the waters. I'm not having my surgery on December 8. It'll probably be closer to Christmas. Does it really matter?

The next day I answer the phone and hear Debra's voice. "Doctor Miller told me about the mix up. He's terribly concerned about you. How are you holding up?"

"I'm fine."

"Doctor Miller told me that you gave up your surgical slot and opted for further testing. I think your choice is wise."

"I want to make an informed decision."

"They're always the best ones."

We chat for a good ten minutes. I hang up the phone feeling I made the right choice. I also feel grateful to have Doctor Miller as my surgeon, and Debra as my liaison. They're a wonderful team.

$\mathcal{A}$S PROMISED, I receive a call back the next day. My ultrasound is scheduled for Thursday. I plan to spend the next few days decorating the house for Christmas. I dig deeply and pull out boxes from the storeroom, boxes I didn't know I had. I lug them upstairs. Packed tight, their sides protrude like gourmands at a buffet.

The morning sun causes the plethora of ornaments to glimmer. I open box after box and wonder where I can put their contents. The task is daunting.

Too much surrounds me. Overwhelmed, I'm motionless. I sit on the floor and stare at the boxes. My anxiety has nothing to do with the ornaments. Not knowing things bothers me. When will I have my surgery? What type of surgery will it be? Does Spike have a twin brother? How in the hell did I get so many ornaments?

I grab a snowman and place it on the sill of the family room window. I conjure Christmas scenes and turn them into reality. Only when pains shoot down my back do I throw myself in a chair and look around. Everywhere I gaze, something stares back at me: Santa, snowmen, dwarfs, a few wise men, and a token baby Jesus. Fa, la, la, la, la. This is going to be a great Christmas. Damn it.

I bake cookies. The freezer fills with Jam Jams, Shortbread, Gingerbread, and Sugar Cookies, essentially every cookie known to man. I stack the overflow on shelves in the garage. I run to the dollar store and buy more containers. Cheating on my gluten free diet is a daily occurrence. I've gained twenty-five pounds since September, if not more. My clothes don't fit. I learn that panties do knot. The sensation leaves me irritable. My gluttonous behaviour has only one positive. The looks I get from acquaintances who somehow find out I have cancer are hilarious.

Their eyes travel up, down, and all around. Their gaze becomes incredulous. "Someone told me that you had breast cancer," they remark in disbelief.

They wait for me to deny the ridiculous tale. How can pudding face have cancer? When I reply: "That's right, I do," nothing is said. They think cancer eats the body. You're not supposed to eat cancer and have an ass twice the size of the one you normally own. Oh well, everyone does things differently. If I could exercise, I might not eat everything in sight, and decorate anything that doesn't move. Then again, I might.

I arrive at the clinic to find myself in the corridor where my journey began. Different faces occupy the same chairs.

I will have an ultrasound without a biopsy. I want the technician to see nothing. I assume it's the best outcome.

I enter the room and make a beehive to the table. I take off my pseudo housecoat, lie down, remove my right arm from the gown, and put it over my head.

The woman doing the ultrasound is not the same woman who did my biopsy. This one is older and not as friendly. Her twisted mouth seems annoyed. She doesn't bother with salutations. She zooms in right away. She concentrates on the ten o'clock position, sighs several times, shows me the mass sitting at twelve o'clock, but fails to find another at ten o'clock. It appears as if it's a false positive.

Eureka, no second tumour! I feel like jumping off the table and doing a jig. Even though I have no idea what a jig entails. It sounds like something you should do when you are overjoyed. Knowing me, I would stub a toe, or knock something down. Luckily, the sour faced technician's demeanour saves me from making a fool of myself and probably breaking something in the process.

Her look of annoyance deepens. It causes lines between her eyes. Head shaking accompanies her sighs. She continues to probe. "Isn't it a good sign that you didn't find something?" I ask.

"It would have been better to see a cyst or some other benign growth." Disgruntled, she continues her search.

"I thought finding naught would be good?" I don't appreciate her bursting my bubble. I try to hold on to it.

Hands on bony hips, she looks at me in annoyance. "No, it's inconclusive. We want to find a benign growth. If I don't find anything, you'll have to have another MRI, with a biopsy."

She continues to press the transducer across my breast. She thrusts harder with every passing second. It feels like an assault. Is she trying to delve through my skin and see what lies underneath? I hold back a scream. She's hurting me. I remain silent. It must be done.

She sighs, and asks: "Why don't you have the mastectomy? I know I would."

Breasts are overrated. They don't stand up to the test of time. Nonetheless, I want to witness them slowly sag. I don't want one severed from my body and thrown in an incinerator.

"It's only a breast," she says.

If a choice is given, whereby I have to cut off an arm, leg, or breast, I'll choose the breast. That said, cutting off any part of your body requires thought. I want to stay whole and, because it is only a breast, some people can't understand that. Would a finger elicit the same reaction? Does the refusal to cut off a breast make one superficial? Is it because breasts are a sexual part of the body? Is my refusal to part with it seen as vanity? I'm not holding onto something entrenched in the sexual allure of women. I'm clinging to a part of myself.

She admits defeat with a grunt. I sigh in relief. Her efforts will surely leave me bruised. The pain radiates throughout my breast. I feel reprimanded.

She's the only hospital employee I don't like. I find her attitude demeaning to women. A woman is not about breasts and an ass, but a woman has breasts and an ass. There's a difference between the two declaratives. Imagine telling someone to throw away a part of their body, as if it is worthless. Who gives her the right to participate in my decision? We're strangers. Would the decision to discard a part come easy, if it was her body?

Her attitude reminds me of a friend's experience. She had breast cancer twenty-five years ago. She decides to have a mastectomy. She opts not to have reconstruction. She and her husband feel comfortable with the decision. She informs her doctor of their choice.

He tries to convince her she's making the wrong choice. Christine doesn't budge. The doctor looks at her in disgust; he points his finger at her. "If you were my wife, I would insist."

Christine is typically outspoken. She's speechless. Later she says: "I wish I would have said: 'Luckily, you're not my husband'."

21

HEN I ARRIVE home from my appointment, a message waits. My MRI is booked for the following day. I shave my legs. I also choose socks appropriate for my age. They're blue, with red bands and Jack Russell dogs frolicking about. Some forms of appropriate, I don't care to follow.

I try to think of something other than cancer. I'm more than a woman living with cancer. It's difficult. Cancer is a bad roommate. It's pushy. It's time consuming. My appointment book fills with cancer's demands. My right breast throbs in pain, restricting activities, reminding me of my roomie.

"Fuck you, roomie, I'm leaving the house without you."

The winter day is sunny. A hint of the departed autumn lives on. It lends a dab of warmth. I squeeze into my old jeans, pull a thick sweatshirt over my head, and run from the house. I don't go far.

I don't have to. My garden is my oasis. Lifeless growth tangles into decomposing knots. The ground is frozen. I can't yank. Instead, I cut away at the dead remains. I work for an hour. I focus on the job and nothing else. When spring comes, my garden will be prepared to welcome the new shoots.

I change into the gowns. A doctor introduces herself. She's a young woman with perfect white teeth and flawless mocha skin. She explains the biopsy procedure. She, not a technician, will oversee the M.R.I.

Her voice is gentle. Her words are not. "We'll take a sample of the abnormality for testing. Since it's difficult to spot, we'll clip it. A mammogram will follow the procedure, to ensure the clip stayed in place. Do you understand?"

I nod. She touches my hand. "Sometimes, if you bleed a lot, the clip slips and we have to do it again. Your breast will probably bruise and there will be pain, but the test will be conclusive. If it is cancer, the clip will guide the surgeon to the site of the mass."

I nod once more. I try to smile. She is kind even though her words are not. I don't understand why they have to clip the tumour. If there is a second mass, my whole breast will be removed. Her logic seems groundless. The clipping reeks of needless torture. I don't bother to voice my opinion.

A patient is accepting ...

I don't feel like superwoman this time around. I feel cold, small, and all alone. As the machine encases my body, the only thing I can do is pray: *Please Lord, let there not be a second cancer.*

I say it repeatedly. I hope to convince Him, by being annoying. You probably can't guess this, but I excel at being trying. I habitually hide this natural ability. *Please Lord, let there not be a second cancer. Please Lord, let there not be a second cancer. Please Lord, let there not be a second cancer. Please Lord, let there not be a second cancer.*

Fine, you don't have a second tumour. Now for God's sake shut up. You're driving Me nuts, you bothersome little twit.

Don't get me wrong. I don't believe in traditional religion. Too many men transcribed the Word, and it reeks of hidden agendas. God's words often ring with the cruelty and narrow mindedness of men. I refuse to believe a higher power is so petty and vindictive. Nonetheless, I do believe in God. Some say people are religious because they seek rewards, while others are spiritual because they seek truth. I believe much of God is lost in man's version of truth. Man replaces answers he does not like with ones that serve him better. Man's meddling does not change God.

Have you ever read Richard Dawkins' book? You know the one, *The God Delusion*. It has a succinct, self-explanatory title so I will not insult you by explaining its major premise. Dawkins speaks of the rational mind pitted against age-old superstitions (Atheist vs. Theist). I enjoyed it immensely but once I'm inside the machine, devoid of outside influences, waiting for a verdict, I choose God. Does fear lead to the decision? Perhaps it has a hand in it. Should I place more worth in the concrete doctors in front of me rather than an entity I can't prove exists? Most would say it's the safer bet. Nonetheless, I choose God. Gut overrides mind, superstition supersedes rationalism, I do what comes natural and don't question why it is so.

I know — yada, yada, yada — what a tirade! I don't care. When you're sick, God enters your life. You may hate him, love him, curse him, or praise him but he is there, regardless if you're roaring, "I don't believe," or trying to strike a deal.

Hey God, you know how I always yell, Jesus Christ, when I'm mad. I promise I won't do it anymore if you take away the second tumour.

Fear courses through my body. It's cold and causes me to shiver. The thought of having a mastectomy is chilling, but I can get through it. I will survive. When something is severed, something fresh always sprouts from the wound.

What causes every nerve to seek information, and grasp at consolation, is the thought of two cancerous growths. Two malignancies make my constitution seem weak and my cancer strong.

I only had one other MRI, but I know something is wrong when a voice informs me they'll be taking further images. I actually say: "Why?"

No one answers me. An MRI provides two-way communications. Why are they ignoring me?

The test continues for an additional five minutes. When the clamour abates, my heart begins to pound. Ultra alert, I feel myself leaving the machine.

I'm on my stomach. I don't face the opening. There's a mirror positioned above my head that allows me to glimpse images of the outside world. Not what is before me, only what is behind me. I can see numerous pairs of legs waiting for me. Why are there so many people in the room? Does it have something to do with the biopsy procedure? Does the freaking procedure require a village to perform it? Is this needle so heavy it needs pairs of arms to hold it up? Given the consent form, I signed, maybe.

As soon as I'm out, I turn myself around and sit up. The pretty doctor sits on a stool beside me. Her pearly teeth glisten. Her body is relaxed. Her reassurance covers me like a shared blanket.

"You won't be having the biopsy," she immediately says.

Relief makes me speechless; I can only stare at her.

"I didn't see anything," she says.

"Does that mean ..."

She doesn't let me finish. Laughing, she throws her arms in the air: "You'll be having a lumpectomy."

I hug her and exclaim: "Thank God."

Only when I feel her body against mine do I realize: *Hey, I'm not a touchy feely kind of person. What the hell am I doing?*

Cancer redesigned me. I'm not familiar with this new person. Cancer took my covert sensitivity and yanked it to the surface. Tears pour from my eyes when something saddens me. I ache over harsh words. I can't pretend to be untouchable any longer. Nonetheless, I'm too happy to care about revealed secrets. I'm sensitive and the pretty doctor doesn't seem to mind my affection. I babble thanks. Accolades burst from the mouths of the technicians. I float out of the room. I passed the test! Yeah!!!

I'm having a lumpectomy. Bring it on! I'm ready. I'm no longer afraid. One cancerous mass is ten times better than two.

22

*W*HEN DOCTOR MILLER calls and suggests we wait until after the New Year to book the surgery, I decline. I want to celebrate the holidays sans cancer. I don't want Spike to join me under the Christmas tree. I don't want him to welcome in the New Year. I want to kick his ass off the premises, as soon as possible.

"I can book you for December twenty-second."

"Perfect," I reply without hesitation. It never occurs to me to consult the family. I assume they will want Spike evicted as much as I do. I'm right. They're behind me one hundred percent.

I'm ashamed to say, I continue to decorate the house. My gaudiness is in overdrive. The house looks garish, but I can't stop myself. I want to keep busy and my family's forced smiles don't sway me into putting away the ornaments.

I have a word I use when (a) someone does a job grudgingly and it doesn't turn out well. It's often the case, when a wife (husband) nags their partner to do something, and they do it half-heartedly, just to get them to shut up; or (b) when embarking on a project, the handyperson completes the task, but unknowingly continues to do more thusly ...

> **Shitifying** the whole thing. The noun is shitification.
> Yes, I shitified the house for the holidays.
> Fa, la, la, la, la, la, la, la, la. I put the Griswolds to shame.
> Christmas lights blind. Riots of reindeer, snowmen and Santas overtake tables. Plush toys occupy dark corners. Button eyes are watchful from above, below, behind and in front. IT IS THE HOLIDAY SEASON!!! And as Clark so astutely put it: We're gonna have the hap hap happiest Christmas since Bing Crosby tap danced with Danny fucking Kaye.

With the surgery scheduled, the question of Christmas day comes up. Are we still going to have everyone over?

"You'll be too weak," my husband says.

"You'll probably be in bed," Madison adds.

"A quiet celebration will be best," Zack says.

Six eyes wait for me to nod in agreement. "No, I don't want that."

"It'll be for the best," Luke says, as he pets my hand.

I snarl: "No! It's my surgery, my rules. Call everyone. Tell them Christmas is on."

I gaze around my cluttered home. I'll pitch the wise men back in the basement. No one likes them anyway. The Santa from my childhood will also return to his cardboard box prison. His beard is yellow, suggesting nicotine addiction and his smile is smarmy, hinting of paedophilia. I prefer the company of friends and family. They always make a situation better. Besides, I'm having a lumpectomy. How bad can it be?

Oddly enough, two days later, my husband proceeds to tell me. How can he be an authority, you ask?

Interesting story! A woman he works with comes into his office one day. I've met the woman at a few office parties, but we're not close. Luke has known her for years, but they share a working relationship. She sits down without preamble. She's a tiny woman, known not to mince words. "I heard your wife has breast cancer."

Luke looks up from his paperwork. "Yes she does," he admits.

The woman holds a bouquet of flowers. "I want you to give these to her." She hands Luke a bunch of daisies, and mums, and baby's breath. "Tell her my thoughts are with her."

Luke takes the offered flowers. "Thank you."

"I had breast cancer eight years ago," the woman says. "I ended up having a lumpectomy with radiation as my treatment."

"That's the treatment my wife is having as well."

"Tell her not to be afraid. It's not that bad. My lumpectomy was not much worse than having the biopsy done. There'll be some pain, but medication will control it. I found the sentinel node biopsy worse than the incision on my breast. She'll have to be careful for a while. No heavy lifting. You'll have to take care of the heavy work."

"I don't have a problem with that."

"Tell her the scars heal nicely. After awhile you can barely see them."

"I'll tell her."

She hands Luke a piece of paper. "This is my phone number. If there is anything, she wants to know, or even if she just wants to talk, tell her to call anytime." She stands. "I consider her to be my sister."

With that, the woman leaves the room.

Isn't it ironic how a malignancy can breed such kindness?

Cancer is despicable. It's a bully. It's self-centred. It's grasping. It's also a teacher. It highlights the uncertainty of tomorrow. Cancer makes strangers friends. Cancer adds depth by illustrating how important life is. Cancer doesn't allow you to take things for granted. It's synonymous with evil, corruption, pestilence, and rot. It's a strong stimulus that elicits negative connotations. Yet once you lance the fear and repulsion, positive qualities remain. Cancer reveals hidden strengths, love, gratitude ... The list is endless. Quite often, when you're facing the worst enemy imaginable, you're at your best, as are the people around you.

23

COME ON DECEMBER 22. Arrive! Quit dragging your feet. Every day prior to surgery seems forty-eight hours long. I want to talk about my surgery in the past tense. I'm sick of it being a part of my future.

Want to feel distress? Tap into the days prior to surgery. Loosen the spigot and sweat, fear, and agitation gush out. The unknown is the most intimidating enemy of all. Reality isn't as shadowy and menacing as one's imagination. The collective consciousness holds prolific caveats.

The day before surgery, I have an appointment with Nuclear Medicine. Since breast cancer often spreads to the lymph nodes under the arm, they demand extra attention.

The lymph nodes are part of your immune system. They help fight infection. You can find them in your neck, groin, and armpits. If you want to understand lymph nodes, think of them as busy little housekeepers. Lymph is a watery liquid that flows between cells. Envision a bucket of water and a mop. It picks up foreign debris (including cancer) and takes it into the lymph node for filtering. The liver then eliminates the typical debris, but not the cancer; it remains in the lymph nodes. About fifteen to thirty percent of women with breast cancer will have cancer in their lymph nodes.

Most women who have a lumpectomy will have a sentinel lymph node biopsy, if the surgeon believes the cancer hasn't spread to the nodes. The surgeon will remove the node that receives lymph drainage from the breast firstly (the dirty water from the bucket). If the cancer has spread, this is where they'll find it. There may be more than one sentinel node. Upon removal, a pathologist examines it. If he or she concludes it's healthy, there's little chance cancer has spread to the remaining lymph nodes. So they remain intact. This procedure is important because it provides information for staging the cancer and it spares women whose cancer hasn't spread to the nodes from having an axillary lymph node dissection, whereby many more nodes are removed. Furthermore, it decreases your risk of lymphedema (an unfortunate side effect of the removal of lymph nodes): arm numbness, difficulty moving your arm and swelling.

Tracers identify the sentinel nodes. Injected into the breast, they then flow through the lymph channels into the underarm. The first tracer uses a small amount of radioactive material. On the day of your surgery, the surgeon will use a hand held Geiger counter to locate the sentinel lymph node during the surgery.

Arriving at the department of Nuclear Medicine, I'm greeted by a young woman who hands me a fresh gown, and asks me to change into it. I lie on the examination table. Once she disinfects my breast, she'll use a small needle to deposit radioactive material through my breast. I'm not scared. It seems straightforward and mundane. Not a big deal. She inserts the needle. She compresses it. The radioactive material begins its journey.

@#!#^!*&^$#*^$#!!!!!

It *is* a big deal. Molten lava courses through my chest. Its path leaves searing pain. Tears spring to my eyes. Let them fall and put out the fire. My body tightens in anguish. I was sucker punched. The hurt is too awful for words.

I remain motionless. A tight ball of pain. The fire abates. My mind restarts. What happened? I look down at my breast. It looks the same. How can something that barely leaves a mark hurt so much?

After fifteen minutes, the technician takes images of my breast and underarm area. She uses a marker to indicate the location of my lymph nodes. I get off the table, dress and drive home.

Once home I make myself a cup of coffee and fire up the computer. I find an interesting article in the ASCO (American Society of Clinical Oncology). They did a study. Twenty patients had the same procedure I did, without topical anaesthetic. They then compared their pain to forty patients who had the same procedure, the difference being the application of a topical anaesthetic. The group without the cream averaged a pain score of 9.08. Zero being no pain and ten being the worst pain you ever felt. (A few of the patients must have been run over by a bus with studded wheels).

Those who had the cream had an average score of 4.15. There's a lesson to learn in these here numbers. If you get the procedure done, tell them to put some anaesthetic cream on your breast before they inject you. If they didn't read the article, point it out to them. Lest you enjoy being tortured.

Quite often, they use a second tracer to pinpoint the sentinel node. It's a blue dye, which they inject during the operation. The dye will leave your body via your kidneys. Your urine and faeces may be blue for a few days. I never asked my doctor if he used a dye, but other woman talked about having a blue nipple. Nothing of mine leaked, seeped, or appeared blue so I assume the molten lava sufficed.

24

*T*HE ALARM SOUNDS. Like a runner who has hit the wall, time finds its second wind and darts to the finish line. Time to shower and drive to the hospital.

Now that the day has arrived, surgery no longer seems like a good idea. Imagine cutting open my skin with a knife! Finding out about my cancer is an even worse idea. Really, who wants to know something like that? Tangled in statistics and probabilities isn't so bad. Definite truths can be such a burden. Standing in front of the mirror, I dry my hair. Dread stares back at me.

A week before my scheduled surgery, a police officer was stabbed in the parking lot of the same hospital I'm going to. Paramedics were at the scene quicker than you can say: "Help me." But they couldn't save him. The assailant severed his jugular. He bled out as trained hospital personnel tried to stop the blood flow. It was a shocking news story. Imagine a police officer murdered as he sat in his car. Now further imagine how it took place in the parking lot of a hospital.

The hospital is a sprawling, brown brick building. It looms. I climb the wide cement steps with Luke. I think back of what took place a week ago. It's irrelevant whether you're on a surgical table, or sitting in your car, parked in front of Emergency, catching up on paper work. Life is bipolar. Tender one minute, ruthless the next. Thinking the worst will drive me mad. With each step I take, I tell myself everything will be fine. Life will shine down on me.

My steps become unhurried. We enter the day surgery facility all the same. I have my medical cards in my hand. They've become as important as a passport. We approach the wicket.

HALT WHO GOES THERE?
I HAND THEM MY PASSPORT.
BREAST CANCER MAY BEGIN PAPERWORK AND THEN ENTER.

Once validated, I let go of Luke's hand, say goodbye, and open the door that separates patients from everyone else.

It's a different world on the other side. A naked man dashes around the lockers. He almost runs me down. He's old and everything hangs and flops as he moves. An orderly attempts to catch him. His fingers brush against the sprinter several times, but he can't grasp him. The elderly man's foggy eyes make it clear he suffers from dementia. He must have been a runner in his younger years, because his legs are strong and sure. He puts up a hell of a fight, but once snagged, becomes docile.

The orderly dresses the man. He then wipes his sweaty brow, and hands me two gowns and a pair of pants. I have the urge to run around the lockers. Dementia bombards the ego, killing reason mercilessly. It tugs at the superego and leaves it in tatters. However, the id, hides in its dark corner. Basic instincts remain intact. The man's dementia feeds misconceptions with faulty data. He breaks protocol effortlessly. However, he's not dim-witted. A light still shines. Who willingly puts themselves under a knife's blade? A human being who understands the necessity of doing what you must. Fine logic but, when the heart beats rapidly, it's difficult to heed.

The pants ground me. The gowns will come off as soon as I'm unconscious, but retaining pants makes the situation bearable.

Most see anaesthesia as the root of their defencelessness. Lying naked on a table makes me feel vulnerable. Clothing is important. Clothes make you more of a person, and less of an object. Clothes are a definite bonus during surgery.

Look, she's wearing pants. She must be of our species.

My cousin was naked on an operating table. She woke up, went home, began changing into her pyjamas, and saw two handprints on her buttocks. Whoever applied the iodine used her as a towel. Just goes to show you, when they disrobe you, they can inadvertently strip humanness from you, along with the clothes. The pants allow me to sustain myself. They are akin to repeating the name of a captive, in hopes of personifying them. Sadly enough, we humans can become cold-hearted, especially when we do something repeatedly. Rather frightening if you think about it.

Once dressed, an orderly wheels me to the day surgery unit. Most of the beds are empty. It's the last day for surgery before the unit closes for the holidays. The nurse on duty introduces herself as Beth, even though her nametag says Elizabeth.

We have plenty of time to talk and I find her entertaining and funny. That is until she brings over the compression stockings. I've blocked them out. Short and muscular, my legs warrant a size large. Making matters worse, my doctor favours the ones that cover your whole leg. Think sexy nurse paraphernalia and now imagine the opposite. These stockings do not slide over your legs. They are unyielding and pitiless. With every tug, they bellow: "My you have big legs."

Difficulties arise as Beth tries to get one over my wide foot. The higher she goes, the worse it gets. Making it pass my calf doesn't seem promising. Beth applies sheer grit and determination. She tugs until they reach my thigh. The battle becomes precarious. Will Beth throw in the towel?

Sorry doctor, it just couldn't be done.

Will they send in reinforcements?

I envision two burly men, a jar of Vaseline, and a derrick. At the count of three ... heave.

Sweat courses through Beth's hair. It drips onto me. I don't say a word. She has the decency not to remark on my Incredible Hulk legs; I don't mention her sweat.

She perseveres, as do I. We pretend a battle isn't taking place. (How fucking embarrassing!!! Bad enough to have stocky legs without having the point drilled home). One final tug and the stocking is on. The second one lies on its side, mocking her. She grabs it and re-enters the battlefield without pause. Ten minutes later, she claims victory. White stockings encase my chunky legs. They feel like sausages whose casings are too tight. Sighing, Beth wipes her oozing forehead. She mumbles something about taking a break as she staggers away.

Some battles don't have an obvious winner. Next time I have surgery I swear I'll take my chances with the blood clots.

Beth returns ten minutes later. She takes my blood pressure. "It's normal," she says, as she pockets the pill she was holding. She looks worn-out. She should sit down.

My annoyance over the stockings shoves my jitters aside. I focus on fixing the problem. I don't dwell on the solution. It's worse to have an ailment without a cure. Surgery is a positive thing! Right. Focus on that. Think happy thoughts. Don't think of your cancer being cut out of you, and then examined in order to see the extent of its damage. Don't think of what they will say, or not say. Concentrate on a victory, achieved one step at a time.

Beth touches my hand. "I just called an orderly to wheel you to the x-ray department. You have to have the pre-operative breast needle localization. They'll tag the lesion to aid the surgeon with its removal."

The procedure is used when the tumour is small.

A tall, gangly, young man releases the brakes of my narrow bed and wheels me down the hallway of the Breast Clinic. Luke joins us on the journey. My eyes dart about. I see Debra. She appears harried. The job of telling women they have cancer never ends. I hope it will one day.

"Good luck, Nan," she calls out when she sees me. Wow, she remembers my name. If I dealt with a sea of patients, names would be lost to me. I can see why Debra is good at her job.

The young orderly manoeuvres down a narrow hallway. His face stiffens as tight as the corner he takes. The bed rattles as he hits the wall.

"Sorry," he says. "Are you all right?"

"I'm fine."

He parks me beside a closed door. Another orderly wheels a patient behind me. Two young women flank her. All three share tallness, slimness, and honey-coloured hair. The recumbent woman appears nervous. Luke says hello and we soon find out our situations are identical. Both of us are having lumpectomies, and both have Dr. Miller as our surgeon. Her surgery will follow mine.

The door opens. The radiologist approaches me.

"I'll let you know how the needle localization goes," I whisper.

I jump off the gurney. Hospital protocol is often senseless. Rules dictate you must be wheeled about. That is, until you reach a doorway that's too narrow to accommodate a wheel chair or a gurney. I follow a short blonde woman into a small cold room.

"Sorry about the temperature," she says.

The cold doesn't bother me. Being uncomfortable is becoming commonplace. Naked, cold, shivering, scared, embarrassed, all have become routine.

The procedure begins easily enough. A mammogram pinpoints the exact location of the tumour. The radiologist numbs my breast with a local analgesic. She then inserts a needle, and threads a small wire through the needle. I feel tugging but no pain. Once done she says: "I have to give you another mammogram to make sure it's in the right position."

She is going to compress my breast after inserting a needle and wire in it. "What, you've got to be kidding?" I squawk.

"Unfortunately not. But, don't worry, the machine won't squeeze hard. You'll barely feel it."

Oddly enough, she's right. It sounds worse than it is.

The position of the tag is correct. She covers it with a paper Dixie cup and then tapes it to my skin. I'm ready to go. I still have an hour before my scheduled surgery. I assume I'll be returning to the Pre-Admission Unit.

Mrs. Adams is still lying on the gurney. Her two daughters flank her like sentries. I have only a few moments to walk upright. I hurry over to her. "Don't worry, it's not that bad."

I don't say any more because the orderly informs me Dr. Miller is waiting. I'm getting in an hour early. Did the person before me cancel? I sincerely hope so.

My orderly tells Luke he can't accompany me any further.

"I'll see you after surgery," Luke says.

I nod and try to smile.

"This is my first day working alone," the orderly admits. "I hope we don't get lost."

"I'm sure we won't."

He begins the trek from the Breast Clinic to the surgical ward. He's so tall he sometimes has to duck as we snake through the tunnels of the old hospital, amid pipes that dart out from the ceiling without obvious rationale. When you lie on a gurney, you have a different perspective of your surroundings. The halls I had travelled seem foreign.

We reach our destination. My hair rustles as he expels a deep breath. "Good luck with the new job. You'll do fine."

"Good luck with the surgery."

The surgical ward consists of multiple beds, cordoned off by curtains. Privacy is a polite illusion. The anaesthesiologist promptly introduces himself. Prior to surgery, I had blood work, and met nurses, and an anaesthesiologist, but my surgery was cancelled. All the people I met worked with whoever took my slot. Strangers surround me.

The anaesthesiologist is tall and thin. Covering his hair is a multi-coloured cap. "Hello, my name is Doctor Stevens. Would you mind sitting up." When I do, he looks directly into my eyes. "Don't worry. I'm very good at what I do. I'll use six needles to inject the pain medication." He touches my back, at six different points to show me the pattern. "It'll block the pain during and after surgery. During surgery, you'll be unconscious."

Sounds good to me.

"Do you typically experience nausea and vomiting after surgery?"

"Always."

"You won't this time."

I don't believe him. They always say that. I usually sneer and call them names, albeit silently, when I wake up and begin to vomit. That's why I ask him to repeat his name.

Doctor Miller opens the curtain and smiles at me. I smile back out of habit, rather than happiness.

Once Doctor Stevens finishes his prep work, he releases the brake, and we journey to the operating room. Smiling individuals throw names at me. I can't catch them. I smile dumbly, as my eyes scan the austere room. I don't take anything in.

Snap, a frozen moment traps me. It freezes the surroundings. Time is elongated. Why are drawn out moments the ones that contain dread, fear and a host of other negative emotions? We open our arms and hearts to happy moments but they always breeze by, leaving just a memory and a smile. Inane conversation takes place, while the anaesthesiologist does his thing. I shiver from the coldness of the room. Surgeons prefer cool environments. I'm in no position to argue. Besides, even though I'm there, I won't be for much longer. The surgeon is doing the work. His comfort is paramount.

My eyes open. I'm in recovery. It's over. Doctor Miller threw Spike from the yard. I won't miss the gnarly beast.

25

*T*HE BEST PART of surgery is waking up afterwards. Not throwing up is a close second. I typically perform a perfect rendition of Linda Blair in the *Exorcist*, but my stomach feels just fine. Lucky, since I forgot the name of my anaesthesiologist. Life is good for the nurses and me. For some reason, hurling patients are never their favourites.

Spotting movement, the nurse trots over and asks if I want ginger ale. I say yes because without it I may never recover. Ginger ale was a big part of my childhood. Some cultures believe in the potency of bull blood, or the healing ability of concoctions of wild flowers. My mother believes in the medicinal benefits of ginger ale. Whenever sickness visits, mother rushes out to acquire the largest bottle offered. The last gulp marks the end of your illness. The nurse hands me the glass and I grasp it greedily.

"How are you feeling?" Nurse Allie asks.

"Fine. I want to go home."

I don't discard the strength of ginger ale but history proves I always ask to go home immediately after surgery. It's reflexive. This is the first time my caregiver doesn't try to talk me into staying.

"Your husband gave me a number to call. He said he would be at his parent's home."

I'm not surprised to hear Luke is at his parent's. They live minutes from the hospital.

Allie calls out: "After I call your husband, I'll be back to help you dress."

She seems anxious to get rid of me and I'm not even vomiting. Maybe vomiting has nothing to do with me not being a favourite patient. Huh. Allie is back with my bag before I finish the ginger ale.

I have the sneaking suspicion her holidays will begin once the ward is empty. It nearly is. For every bed with a patient in it, four beds are unoccupied. People don't want surgery near Christmas, and surgeons don't want to perform them. I'm glad I squeaked in, especially now that it's over.

The menu in recovery is basic. They serve toast.

"I'm gluten intolerant."

"Crackers then?"

"No thanks."

"You should eat something."

I'm not hungry but she looks determined to feed me. I suspect she's intent on ensuring I have enough energy to make it out the door.

"I have dried mango slices in the side pocket of my bag. If you don't mind getting them."

Her smile is quick and sure. "I don't mind at all."

When Luke arrives, I'm dressed and waiting to leave. He talks of the conversation we had after my surgery. I supposedly fell asleep in mid sentence. I don't remember any of it. The nurse shoed him away with assurances I'd sleep for hours. Less than an hour later, I'm awake and annoyed. Why does it take him so long to retrieve me? Turns out, I'm ready before the pharmacy can fill my prescription.

I sit quietly in the car and dream of having coffee. As soon as we arrive home, I ask Luke to prepare one. His face scrunches up. "I don't know if you should have one. You just had surgery."

"But I'm home now, so hospital rules no longer apply."

"It was cancer surgery."

"It was day surgery. I want a coffee."

He looks at the coffee maker but makes no move to get up. I roll my eyes. "I was awake within two hours of having surgery. I was then dressed to go home. Shortly after, I was walking. I deserve a coffee."

"I'll make you your coffee, but then you're off to bed."

I nod with happiness.

The coffee tastes heavenly, but the cup feels heavy in my hand. I don't argue when Luke leads me to bed. The smell of chicken cooking wakes me. I'm starving. I hurry out of bed and sit in my regular spot at the dinner table before anyone can ask if I need assistance.

Luke places the plate before me. I attack it with the relish displayed by a lion clutching an antelope. My family stares at me in horror. What? I'm hungry!

After dinner, we talk and watch Christmas specials on television. When the children were young, I claimed to watch the animated specials with them. There came a time when I had to fess up. I watch them because I enjoy them. I never grow tired of the Grinch, even though I can recite it by heart. I can feel eyes watch me throughout the evening. What are they expecting? Swooning and moaning?

When it's time for bed, I glance down at my bandages, relieved I don't have to see what's underneath. The breast I knew so well is gone. What takes its place is new and not improved. Oh well, getting rid of Spike is all that matters.

๑ 26 ๑

HAVING SURGERY AND asking people to join you for dinner is akin to having the flu, accompanied by runny green mucus oozing from your nose, and fever blisters that surround your mouth, and the offering of a kiss.

"No, no, no, it's alright, you don't have to," is the immediate response.

No one wants to come to our home for Christmas. They decide it'll be too much for me. I need my rest. It takes numerous calls to assure the family we want them over. It's easier to have them come to me, rather than me going to them. Spending Christmas not surrounded by family is not an option. Reluctantly, they agree, but insist they'll bring food. I'm not to do anything but be my charming self. Okay, they didn't say that. I'm never accused of being charming. I don't know why.

My mother is coming over on the twenty-fourth to cook the Christmas Eve meal and prepare the turkey and stuffing for the following day. She insists she wants to do her fair share, which in reality is a lot more than just fair. She loves to feed people and I have to point out several times that others are bringing food too.

We have a quiet December 24, which is exactly how I like it. She's the prelude to her rambunctious sister. I appreciate her taciturn spirit because Christmas is always frantic. We watch *Christmas Vacation* and it's like visiting old friends. That movie always makes me happy. How can it not? They're totally nuts. We laugh like fools and then head off to bed.

On Christmas day, everyone hurries to shower and dress in his or her finest. Following surgery, I can't bathe for five days. Do the math. There's no shower, no deodorant, no powder, and no perfume for Christmas. I wash my hair and sponge bathe. I can only wash one armpit. The incision under my arm burns because I sweat. There, I said it. I don't perspire. I sweat — sometimes profusely. When I tell my surgeon my theory of an open cut, burning pain and dripping sweat, he pretends not to hear me.

It feels as if battery acid is dousing my incision. The pain is raw and constant. It prompts me to think of a solution. Plato said necessity is the mother of invention. Truer words cannot be spoken. But who's the daddy? Pain is a good one. He propels you into action. You don't procrastinate when he's around.

Active people buy form fitting moisture wicking tees to absorb sweat and keep the body dry. My son is a workout junkie. He has three under armour tees. I borrow one and the burning pain goes away. I also make myself a little pillow. My breast hurts whenever I sleep on my stomach, which I always do, regardless of intentions. The tiny feather pillow is softer than my mattress. The complaining boob is satisfied and wakes up refreshed. The pillow is also useful when my sentinel biopsy incision hurts. I place it under my arm and it stops friction.

Our guests arrive en masse, arms laden with presents and food. My husband and children hurry to the door to greet them. Cane, our black lab, takes centre stage. He smells each of them, gets a whiff of the ham and begins to drool. I stand away from the door since the air rushing in is cold and biting.

The people entering our home look like our family members, but they're not. They're zombies. Thirteen people are in the house and you can hear the dog fart. What happened to the loud mouth sister? She's unnaturally silent. It's downright eerie.

When my niece exclaims: "You look good," in an amazed manner, I understand. They believe they'll be eating over a half-dead body.

Don't mind me, enjoy yourselves. Ahh, the pain, the horrible pain! No, no, don't touch that, it's not cranberries, my stitches ripped open.

"I feel fine," I announce.

"You do look good," Nadia says.

"I can't believe you're dressed," Caitlin admits.

"Why wouldn't I be? It's Christmas and I feel fine."

I'm glad I wore makeup and a blouse with ruffles. I look fine because I am fine. The cancer is gone and the pain medication is working. The incision is bothersome, but the knowledge of being cancer free is liberating. I escaped cancer's grip. What more can I ask for?

Once that silliness is over, we celebrate Christmas. I can't drink the wine. Doctors frown upon mixing booze and hydromorphone. I don't care. I don't need spirits to be happy.

Remember when I told you that some people didn't acknowledge my disease. One of them is my brother-in-law. He speaks to others about my predicament. He tells them I'm too young to face such an adversary. He expresses anger, but never mentions the C word to me. Funny. Before having cancer I thought the unspeakable C word was *cunt*. Live and learn. Rudeness and disrespect pales along side of deadly.

On Christmas day when the meal is over, I see my brother-in-law in the kitchen. He's wearing my apron as he polishes the counter and helps load the dishwasher.

EW YEAR'S EVE is a quiet affair. I can't party and that's fine. No one is in the mood to celebrate.

We woke up to realize Cane had a stroke during the night. He can't walk, and it looks as if we will have to euthanize him. Really, can things get any worse? He's fourteen and we should be grateful for the years we've had him. We're not. We love him and don't want to say goodbye. His legs can't move. His eyes are alert. He's happy when someone pets him, and excited when you bring him his food bowl. Poor Cane looks puzzled. He appears encouraged when we're near.

We google and find an article which explains the paralysis might not be permanent. Cane's pleading look convinces us to give him time to recover.

Every four hours Luke carries the ninety-pound dog outside to do his business. Friends come over and, when they see Luke carrying Cane, you can see they think he's crazy. I don't think he's crazy. I love him for it.

My daughter breaks up with her boyfriend. Her sobs accompany the dog's moans. Hers was not an easy decision. They dated for six years. We feel as if a family member was yanked from us. The holidays make the atmosphere even more hellish. Misery amplifies when joy is compulsory and it's lacking.

Everything is changing, and not for the better. We're awaiting the pathology report. I did well in, and after surgery, but we don't know anything about the cancer. Was it slow growing, or fast? Mean or timid? Are the nodes as clean as we expect them to be? We won't find out until January 6. I'm afraid to be hopeful.

We're not a joyful household. None of us sees midnight. New Year's Eve exemplifies bleakness when things are calamitous.

PARTY!!!!

Piss off.

*J*ANUARY SIXTH ARRIVES. The day of truth. I'll learn more about my little friend. It's also the day our family dog begins to walk. Surely, a good sign.

Poor old Cane holds his head crooked, as if waiting for an answer to a puzzling question. However, he can walk. His steps are slow but sure.

I sympathize with Cane. Sickness barges in and takes control from you. You're at its mercy. It fills your appointment books. Sickness frightens, disheartens, clings tightly, or abandons you. I hope it is done with Cane and me. I want our lives to be our own again.

Doctor Miller enters the conference room, sits at the round conference table and smiles. He has the pathology report in his hand.

"Did you enjoy your holidays?" I ask.

His eyebrows rise. "They were very nice." He looks quizzical. I guess one doesn't expect niceties at such a time.

We quickly get down to business. Doctor Miller heads to the back page of the report, aptly named "Diagnosis". Previous pages talk about clinical information, procedures preformed to the specimen, gross description, and microscopic description.

"It was invasive carcinoma as suspected. Immohistochemical studies show it's positive for E-cadherin." He finds my eyes. "That shows a better prognosis. The carcinoma is the NOS type." My brow knits. "That means not otherwise specified. Eighty percent of cancers fall in this category. Your Bloom Richardson score is six out of nine. Do you know what that means?"

I know about the Bloom Richardson scale. Pathologists scrutinize three features when determining a cancer's grade: the frequency of cell mitosis (rate of cell division), tubule formation (percentage of cancer composed of tubular structures), and nuclear pleomorphism (change in cell size and uniformity). Each of these variables is allotted a score ranging from 1 to 3 (1 indicating slower cell growth and 3 indicating faster cell growth). The scores of each of the cells' features are then added for a final sum that will vary between 3 to 9. It's a grading system which determines how aggressive the cancer is. It also quantifies how the tumour looks. My score of six is middle ground.

"Not the best prognosis, or the worst," I say. "A medium prognosis."

"Correct," he replies. "In the centre of the largest tumour we found a hematoma. (A semisolid mass of blood in the tumour, caused by injury). It must have been caused by the biopsy you had done."

The results explain the need for a hot compress. Only two percent of biopsies result in hematomas.

Doctor Miller looks down at the papers before him. Why did he specify it was found in the largest tumour? Was there more than one growth? Before I can ask, he continues.

"No vascular invasion was identified. That means that there was no cancer invading blood and lymphatic vessels. There was also no perineural invasion. By that I mean cancer growing around nerves."

"That's all good, right?"

"Very good but the cancer was multifocal. Two foci of invasive carcinoma were identified. The largest was stage pT2. The smallest focus measured microscopically at 1.5 mm in diameter. We found it in the deep-inked surface. In other words, past the margin I cut around the tumour. Deeper in the chest, where it could not be reached by a scalpel."

Two, two, two for the price of one. Shit. He downplays the finding of the second foci but I notice when he speaks of my treatment he no longer says lumpectomy with radiation. It's now lumpectomy, radiation, and possibly chemotherapy. When we're done, he says the radiation oncologist and medical oncologist will call within a week.

29

O N THE RIDE home, I keep looking at the pathology report. "It could have been worse," I conclude.

"It could have been better," Luke mutters.

"I would have preferred a lower score on the Bloom Richardson scale."

"A three would have been nice."

"Even a five, at least I would have squeezed into the best category. Instead of being stuck in the middle. It's the stupid tubule score that screwed me." I had a 3/3 on tubule formation, the worst score because less than ten percent of the lesion was composed of tubular structures. I feel as if I failed a large section of an exam.

"I didn't like the mention of a second foci," Luke remarks.

"No, but Doctor Miller said that the sample could have folded."

"Could have, isn't very specific.

Cancer is ambiguous. Definitive conclusions are nonexistent. There are so many variables involved that it's impossible to have a definite diagnosis. Even when everything goes well, you worry about a reoccurrence. Most reoccurrences take place in the second year. So over is not really over. Physically escorted from the yard, Spike might decide to return. He might come back bigger and stronger than before. He might even bring friends. It's an agonizing thought. One I refuse to dwell on. I'm not going to spend two years holding my breath. To hell with it. Whatever happens, happens. Worrying will not help, so why bother.

"Let's stop at the fruit store and buy some persimmons?" I say.

"Let's get some bananas too."

Life will go on, as it always does. Life doesn't keep scores. Life allows losers to play. You stay in the game, even though you're beaten. Life ends when life ends. I hate my scores. I hate the uncertainty the report disclosed. I hate how cancer is still a part of my life.

I went under the knife to get it cut out. Did a little part stay behind?

"*H*ELLO, MY NAME is Doctor Justin Stewart."
Luke turns his head and doesn't like what he sees.
"How old are you?" he asks.

Doctor Stewart evades the question. His stance is tense as he speaks of his years of experience in his chosen field.

It takes many years of education to be a radiation oncologist. Most have a Bachelor of Science degree, followed by four years of medical school. A year of internship is required before entering residency graduate education, which usually takes about four years. Thusly even your young doctors are not very young. Unless you pit them against the white haired persona we expect them to be. My doctor has brown hair, glasses, and an unlined face.

Good doctor = years of experience.
Bad doctor = fresh graduate.

I find the computation lacking. I don't mind young. Enthusiasm and the need to prove oneself can spur first-class treatment. Besides, Doctor Stewart seems serious and conscientious. He's familiar with my case and, after doing an examination, explains my treatment to me.

"There is the possibility of chemotherapy. I assume you'll be having six rounds of chemotherapy, but your medical oncologist will decide this. You'll also be receiving twenty-three fractions of radiation, and brachytherapy."

Chemotherapy is a concoction of drugs given intravenously. Doctor Stewart explains how treatment is given every three weeks. My medical oncologist will decide on what drugs and what timetable. Radiation begins approximately four and a half weeks after chemotherapy. Radiation entails daily visits, Monday to Friday.

"Exactly what is brachytherapy?" I ask.

"In your case it'll be a boost to ensure the cancer deep in your chest is eradicated. Brachytherapy treats the cancer with a high total dose of radiation in a concentrated area for a short period of time. It's especially effective for cancers that are hard to reach. With this therapy, sealed radioactive sources are placed in the body. Needles will be surgically implanted whereby radioactive seeds will course through."

"I see," I say, unaware that *needle* doesn't accurately describe the skewers they plunge into your chest.

"I'm also going to call Doctor Miller and ask if further surgery is warranted."

Further surgery? Is my boob back on the table? Is it going to get whacked this time around? I don't bother asking. I'll find out soon enough. I'm getting tired of hearing how everything is going fine. Then suddenly the situation turns ominous, only to return to fine once again. Besides, I'm sure Doctor Miller will not recommend further surgery. During our meeting, he mentioned he couldn't reach the second foci without flaying me. A mastectomy would get rid of the breast, but it wouldn't reach the cancer.

I have to give the young doctor credit. I arrive home to a ringing telephone.

"Doctor Miller and I discussed your case. We concluded there will be no further surgery."

Bonus points for punctuality. He didn't give me enough time to worry about additional surgery.

a MEDICAL ONCOLOGIST specializes in diagnosing and treating cancer using hormonal therapy, chemotherapy, and biological therapy. When I meet Doctor Lindsey, I'm pleased. He's a laid-back individual whose presence makes me feel comfortable. I appreciate how he sits down beside me, paper in hand, and makes notes I can keep, as he explains my situation. Facts overwhelm, when disposed in heaps. Add an emotional component and the brain muddies further.

"We use biomarkers (indicators, in terms of characteristics that can't be seen under a microscope, but can be measured by molecular tests) to determine how a tumour will behave. It helps us predict what treatment will be beneficial and it aids us in determining the prognosis. Your tumour is sensitive to oestrogen and progesterone."

"Is that good?"

"Yes. Tumours sensitive to hormones are generally slower growing and have a better prognosis than tumours that are not. Because of this sensitivity, we can treat your cancer with a hormone blocking therapy. Since your tumour has the receptors to hormones, I'll prescribe tamoxifen. It blocks the oestrogen receptor in the breast, and in the metastatic cancer cells, preventing oestrogen from reaching them."

"Does that mean that my body will stop producing oestrogen?"

"No, it's more complicated than that. What it does is stimulate the ovaries to make more oestrogen in other organs such as the uterus and bone." His eyes look grave. "That's why you will be more susceptible to uterine cancer and blood clots. However, it has its benefits. You'll have increased bone mass and lower cholesterol."

Lowering the cholesterol is good, especially with my history, but uterine cancer and blood clots I can do without, thank you very much. I don't bother asking about the statistics of the risk factors. The threat of reoccurrence of breast cancer warrants the risk, or he wouldn't prescribe it. Instead, I ask: "How long will I have to take tamoxifen?"

"The most effective duration is five years."

'Why not longer?"

"The longer a woman takes it, the greater the benefit, but only up to five years. We once believed cessation of the drug would wake up sleeping cancer cells. Studies proved the line of thinking incorrect. Benefits persist long after the drug is discontinued. If you take the drug for even one year, the benefits last for at least twenty-one years. To answer your question, recent studies have shown that, if you take tamoxifen longer than five years, the cells can become resistant to it."

Doctor Lindsey's statistics deal with survival, rather than reoccurrence. He bases the prognosis on survival estimates for ten years. Age and the risk of breast cancer death are calculated, with and without adjuvant therapy. My odds of survival increased to 79.9% because I've had surgery to remove the tumour. Tamoxifen increases it to 84%. Chemotherapy will increase my odds to 86%.

He then proceeds to explain the effects of each treatment. "If you're at an age where you'll soon enter natural menopause (I am), tamoxifen can nudge you into menopause sooner. If not, your menstruation will resume with the cessation of the medication. Women taking tamoxifen usually experience hot flashes, but as I've already mentioned, there's a lowering of cholesterol. Unfortunately, because of the increase of blood clots and uterine cancer, monitoring and a yearly pap test is mandatory. When everything is considered, the advantages outweigh the negatives. Chemotherapy has many side effects. If you decide you want chemotherapy, you'll have three treatments, every twenty-one days. (I note right off, he's saying I'll decide.) You'll experience hair loss, possibly nausea, infections, sore mouth, bone pain and chemo brain. There's a small chance of developing leukemia and damage to the heart is possible."

Tamoxifen is a no brainer. But chemo ...

"That's a lot of side effects for a two percent difference," I remark. Four percent would leave me thinking about it. I would have done it, had it been five percent but two percent ...

"When you consider the benefits of chemotherapy, you have to understand it reduces the risk by about a third. Therefore the higher the risk, the more beneficial chemotherapy is."

"I'm not doing it. Two percent is not a high enough gain. Not when you consider all the things that can go wrong."

"Don't make a hasty decision. Think about it. I'll set up another appointment for you. Weigh your options and then let me know what your decision is after you've thought about it."

I never saw chemo as an option. Too much at stake for too small a reward. I'm surprised when Luke is not like-minded.

"I would do it even if it was one percent," he says when we're alone in the car. "Every little bit helps."

My body will have to endure the treatment. Therefore, it's my choice. Luke's rationale is straightforward. Anything that increases the odds in your favour is worth it. He doesn't consider all the things that can go wrong. Chemotherapy is beneficial, but it's a toll on your body. It'll put me at risk for other diseases and infections. I can increase my odds, slightly, but end up with leukemia or heart disease.

Luke eventually agrees with my decision but I know, if he faced the same situation, he would have taken the chemo. Everybody has a magic number. Luke's was one. Mine was five.

Two weeks pass. I meet with Doctor Lindsey to turn down chemo again. He doesn't try to talk me out of it. I think we're like-minded about the benefits in my particular case. Or perhaps I only convince myself that we are.

Having refused chemo, I will begin radiation.

32

*D*OCTOR STEWART DETERMINES I'll have twenty-three daily treatments. It will begin in two weeks. There's no discussion, no choice. As soon as I chose to have a lumpectomy, rather than a mastectomy, radiation became compulsory.

I'll have a bone and chest scan before getting myself permanently tattooed. I assume my doctor is running the tests to screen for metastatic disease. I don't ask, and he doesn't explain. Metastasis is something I don't want to discuss. For it's the most daunting of words. It means the cancer has spread from the original tumour to other parts of the body. The spread occurs when microscopic bunches of cells are transported by the blood or lymph. The primary treatment for cancer is surgery. You can't cut out cancer that has metastasized if it's too widespread.

I don't scare easy. I can deal with a cancerous tumour. Spike stole a piece of my breast. I'm not happy about it. I'm happy it's over.

Is it over? Could Spike have had a litter before eviction? Has my world gone to the dogs? If each takes a piece of me, there might not be enough of me left to fight back. I take the requisition forms. They frighten me.

The bone scan is important because, in twenty-five percent of breast cancer cases, the bones are the first site they detect metastatic disease.

The scan is a nuclear medicine test because the technician injects a low level of radioactive particles into your vein (painless). After the injection, you have to wait a few hours for the test to begin. You must allow your bones to pick up the radioactive particles. My appointment is for seven o'clock on Monday morning. After the injection, I go home and return two hours later. I lie on a narrow table. A machine hovers over me. It takes a picture of my skeleton. In areas where the bone is actively metabolizing, the radioactive particles show up stronger, than static areas. The test is trouble-free, except when it scans my head and I can't see. The visual deprivation leads to thinking ...

Everyone believes cancer is the dirtiest of words, but anyone in the know recognizes metastasis as the foulest of all words. It's the sound one hears when hope dies.

Humans are supposedly the only species to understand death. As a human, I feel I must qualify that statement. The human brain understands death. Death is the cessation of all biological functions that sustain a living organism. It's easy enough to comprehend. No heartbeat, no brain activity, flat lines, death.

THE END???

Most human hearts and minds do not understand death.

YOU CANNOT TAKE A LOVED ONE AWAY FOREVER!

I CANNOT CEASE TO LIVE. LIFE IS TRUTH AND TRUTH MUST EXIST TO BE VALID!

Religion pierces fear, releasing the passage to resurrection, redemption, and reunion.

Death pushes, as surely as birth. You accept it, because you must. You reinvent it, because you can.

Does stomping on religion prove you're fearless? Or is it an illustration of the narrowness of thoughts?

The world was once flat. If one journeyed too far, one plunged into nothingness. We journey further than our predecessors did, yet boundaries still exist. Death is a cessation, rather than a continuance into the unknown. Our world remains absolute. Level, measurable, comprehensible. Conceptions change, but underlying principles do not.

The scan is over. Thoughts recede. I can see again ...

The following day I have a chest scan to ensure the cancer has not spread to my lungs. The tests are frightening because if I receive a call back, I'll die, figuratively and perhaps literally. It's unnerving.

The tests conclude. The telephone does not peal. I can breathe once again.

The next step is the planning session at the radiation department. It takes an hour. I find myself in a radiation simulator. It's comparable to a radiation machine but doesn't emit radiation. (Instead it uses the same energy as an X ray machine.) I make myself comfortable. The position I'm in will be the same one used for my twenty-three treatments. They take measurements. They map my body, taking into account where organs are in relation to one another. I'm tattooed. Five blue dots will aid in my radiation therapy by serving as markers. They'll help technicians position me properly. They'll also tell any future oncologist where I've been radiated, since you can only radiate an area once. Radiation doesn't seem like something you could ever forget. Blue dots or not. The dots are the size of a freckle. They'll remain on my skin for the rest of my life. One more souvenir of breast cancer.

A friend of mine loves tattoos and has three of them. Gravity makes me leery about the prudence of getting a tattoo. Imagine a cute spider dangling from a web. Imagine the day you wake up and can't find the spider. Ouch! Mine are only little blue dots. It didn't hurt and I resign myself to them. I want optimum treatment and, if blue dots assist in my sessions, I won't complain. Much.

They take a photograph of me in a johnny. With every treatment, they match the person lying on the table with the photo. Since treatment is individualized, they have to make sure they're radiating the right person. It's a safety measure. Mistakes must have happened in the past, or they wouldn't employ the measures.

a SNOWSTORM HITS the city the day the local buses go on strike. I look out the window and see only whiteness. As luck would have it, my radiation therapy begins that day.

I'm never late for anything, regardless of how meaningless it is. I see lateness as a statement: *I'm more important than you are. My needs come before yours.*

It's a twenty-minute ride to the hospital. I give myself an hour. The bus strike ensures every car in the city is on the road. The snowstorm guarantees we creep. At one point, it looks as if I'll actually arrive on time. Suddenly everything stops. We do not move. Not an inch, for at least five minutes. We then advance so slowly I almost feel I should shut down the engine. I'm blocks from the hospital. Walking would be quicker, but you can't abandon your vehicle. Running out of curse words, I listen to the radio.

My head is down when I take the elevator to the basement. My cheeks are red when I check in at the desk and admit my appointment was for nine o'clock. It's nine thirty, but the woman understands the delays. Besides, I have cancer. No one ever gets mad at me. It was somewhat nifty at first but it gets tiresome.

The smiling, bubbly receptionist hands me a card. It specifies my appointment times for the week. I had asked for morning appointments. They're all for 7 o'clock, except for Friday. I get to sleep in: 7:15.

"You have to swipe the card on every visit. It tells the computer and the people who look at the computer you have arrived." She gets up and says: "Follow me. I'll introduce you to your treatment nurse."

The treatment nurse is small, barely five feet tall. She has the face of Casey, Mr. Dressup's sidekick.

"I'll start by explaining the effects of radiation, beginning with the worst one: Fatigue. Your body will be using a lot of energy to heal itself. Even if you sleep well, you may still feel exhausted. Tell us if you cannot perform your daily tasks."

I don't sleep well, prior to starting radiation. I promise to keep her informed.

"Radiation also affects your skin. It can look sunburned or tanned. It could become swollen and sore. Peeling and blistering can also happen. Your breast could also change size, or shape, and may feel firmer. I recommend that you buy calendula cream. During treatment, don't use creams, powders, perfumes, deodorants, body oils, ointments, ice packs or heat packs unless approved by someone on my team. Always express any concerns you have. It's important to communicate."

"A friend of mine bought me an aloe plant. Can I use that?"

"Yes, aloe is very good. Any other questions?"

"No."

"Okay then, let's begin."

We walk into a darkened room. The table seizes my attention. It's narrow, like a surgical table. A large radiation machine looms to one side. A female technician flanks each side of the table. They smile, introduce themselves, and then ask me to lie down and assume the position: bared breasts, right arm over my head. Ho-hum.

"We're going to position you," one of them says. "Please don't help us." She smiles, but her firm tone highlights her request.

"You want me to act like a sack of potatoes?"

"Pretty much."

It seems like a simple request. Once they punch my particulars into the computer, a green beam lights my chest with a triangulated graph. My photograph is perched on the side of the computer console, looking thoughtful. No one has volunteered to take my place, so yes here I am.

They begin positioning me, using my pant loops to move me a little to the right, a little to the left. Each technician matches the blue dots on her side to the lines of the graph.

Acting like a sack of potatoes sounds easier than it is. When they hoist me, I repeatedly assist them, which is not helping them at all. I cause them to overshoot their target. I'm a bad sack. They tell me twice to quit HELPING.

It takes them ten minutes to line me up. They turn to leave the room and I ... sneeze. My hand automatically covers my mouth.

They both look at me. Nothing is said, but their frustration bounds across the room and surrounds me. I was late for my appointment and I'm a rotten squirmy sack. I'm a bad patient, but since I have cancer, one of them forces her tight lips into a smile and says: "Let's begin again."

The taller of the two grabs hold of my pant loop. "Remember, don't help us, and don't move."

I play dead. A technician painted the ceiling. The sea scene depicts clown fish swimming around coral. I will my body not to twitch, sneeze, itch, or do anything disruptive. Look at the clown fish and pretend you're on the ocean's floor. You're a locked trunk, incapable of movement.

Once they leave the room, the machine begins to move. It's no longer to the right of me. It's over me. Pulsating noises fill the room. Then the noise abruptly stops. It deepens the silence. The light of the camera twinkles, enabling the technicians to see me.

To watch someone being radiated must be boring. Reality television at its worst. It would only be exciting if someone freaks out. I might sneeze and move about, but I'm calm and motionless in the dark, even with a machine looming over me.

After a few seconds, the machine approaches me from a different angle. It's now to the right of me. A hum infuses the room, then silence. I hear a door open. The technician appears.

"It's over. You can get dressed and go home."

Before she can assist me, I'm off the table.

"See you tomorrow," she says with a smile.

Tomorrow, and the day after that, and the day after that. It seems endless and disheartening when you begin your journey.

I just get home when the doorbell sounds. The dogs bark. I lurch to the door because they're underfoot. I'm not expecting visitors and wonder whom it can be. I see a man's legs, and arms, through the glass. Instead of a head, I see a bouquet of flowers.

"Are you Nancy Burns?" flower head asks.

"I am."

He hands me the bouquet and is halfway down the stairs when he says: "Have a nice day."

"You too, flowerhead," I say, once the front door closes firmly and he's sitting in his truck.

I hurry to the kitchen and rip the covering off the bouquet. Twelve newly opened white tulips peek up at me. Branches of pine provide a green background, giving the arrangement a winter motif. A silver ribbon tied around the vase makes it look dazzling. I find the card:

Thinking of you, wishing you well. Love Nadia and Rob.

Flowers don't last forever. Sentiments do. The arrival of the bouquet is timely. I will never forget my niece's kindness. She lives hours away. The flowers feel like a hug. Thanks Nad. Thanks Rob.

34

I GET OUT of bed at five thirty, drag myself to the coffee maker. I arrive for my appointment twenty-five minutes early. Traffic is better and the snowstorm is a distant memory. I park on a side street to avoid giving my soul to the parking attendant at the hospital.

I enter the hospital through the side doors. I follow the signs that say, Cancer Clinic. Blue dots painted on the floor prompt me to stay on path. They indicate where to turn, or go straight. They lead me through doors and bypass others. The blue dots guide my destiny.

Tests confirmed I had cancer. A surgeon removed my cancer. Nonetheless, it feels frightening to follow the blue dots. In my pre-cancer days, I always thought I would follow the yellow dots to the Heart Institute. I always imagined myself being older than I am now.

This must be a joke. My family's medical history practically guarantees I'll die from heart disease. At thirty years of age, I forced my doctor to test my cholesterol. She didn't see the need, given my age, gender, weight and lifestyle. When the results came back she said: "It's not a question of if you're going to have a heart attack, but when."

It's not a shock. Everyone on my father's side dies from thrombosis at an early age. They clutch their chest and are dead before they hit the floor. Being an impatient sort, I have to admire how the killer doesn't dawdle. I could do without premature death, but Fortuna snatches many significant choices. Why did she feel she had to send another serial killer after me? Especially since both are her best assassins. Seems like overkill.

The blue dots on the floor are larger versions of the blue dots tattooed on my chest. I'm clearly marked to follow those dots. Nonetheless, it feels odd. I don't know why.

I swipe my card, change, and go to the waiting room. A woman wearing a blonde wig and dressed in the double hospital gowns is reading a magazine. I draw closer and note the drawn on eyebrows, the lack of eyelashes. She has had chemo. She looks up when I enter the room.

"Hi," I mumble.

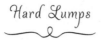

"Hi." Her eyes are inquisitive. "Never saw you before. Just starting out?"

"Yeah. Only my second treatment."

"My fifth."

"Who's your doctor?"

"Abul. And you?"

"Stewart."

"Breast cancer?"

"Yeah, stage 2a."

"No chemo?"

"No."

"Lucky. I was stage three."

"Nodes involved?"

"No, but the tumour was large."

"You must be glad that it's drawing to an end?"

Her painted on eyebrows furrow. "I can't envision it being over. I've been a patient for so long, I can't remember the person I once was. It'll be nice to get to know her again."

I wonder if that person still exists. There is life after cancer, but is it the same life?

"You had a rough go at it?" I ask. She is a big woman, tall and wide but she seems frail.

"Chemo was bad. After the fifth session, I was rushed to the hospital with fever and dementia. They ran tests and thought I had AIDS. The chemo took out my immune system. I was supposed to go for six rounds before surgery, but they said the sixth one would kill me. We had to wait for surgery, until they brought my blood count up."

"Darcy O'Grady," the technician calls out.

Darcy grabs a pink purse that has a large leather bow adorning it. Her feet wear pink shoes that match the purse in colour and style. They too have a bow. She rises and says: "See ya."

I do see her and she sees me. Cancer is akin to joining a club. You don't ask to join, but once you're in the ranks, it's forever. Differences that once existed are no longer important. You share one commonality, but it is so monumental, it transcends everything else. As the odyssey unwinds, you knot together as you share one goal. We all want to be well. We never want to hear a doctor solemnly tell us that we have cancer, ever again. Is it asking too much?

35

*G*OING TO THE hospital for radiation every day is boring, annoying, exhausting, and time consuming. Seeing the same women daily is not any of the above. Familiar faces make the experience easier. Within a week, I know who's in the dressing room beside me, even though I can't see them.

Beverly never closes her locker. She always wears a green coat with a fur collar. If you hear humming, it's Martha. Old show tunes are her favourite. Barbra brings knitting with her. When you spot yarn dangling, Barbra is beside you. Each woman makes her presence known, in her own special ways.

I change into my double gowns, leave the cubicle, and nearly run into Connie. She's frowning at her reflection in the mirror, outside the change rooms.

"Have you noticed most of the women have blonde wigs, and draw eyebrows using a light honey colour?" she asks.

Whenever you look up, at least four out of five women wear short-tussled blonde wigs, and each appears to share the same eyebrow pencil. "I never noticed," I say, lying. I never thought my thick shiny hair and bushy eyebrows would make me feel guilty.

Connie is the average age for the women I meet in the radiation department: late sixties or early seventies. She's very sensitive about her appearance. I try to be careful when I talk to her. I often fear my blunt nature bulldozes my intentions.

She continues to frown at her image. "I'll be so glad when my eyelashes grow back. In some ways not having eyelashes is worse than losing the hair on my head."

"They'll grow back soon enough," I assure her.

She sighs and turns away from the mirror. "Not soon enough."

Women and their looks, why are we so vain?

Years ago, I sat in a doctor's waiting room. I reached for a magazine and read an article that stayed with me, because I thought it was ridiculous.

Aimed at flat-chested women, it promises to bestow the appearance of breasts. It's titled something witty like: How to go from flat to fab. It implies flat is not fabulous. A push up bra is obligatory. Creating a cleavage by using various makeup techniques is a must.

I imagine scenarios where your cleavage runs, staining your clothes. I'm so embarrassed my shirt is blushing!!!

Joking aside, I can't see why women have to use makeup to create a cleavage. What next? We wax nearly every part of our body. News flash: one of the characteristics of a mammal is having fur or hair. The definition goes on to say that not all mammals keep their fur or hair throughout their lifespan. They must mean us women. Really, we should band together and fess up: *Yes, I have hairy legs, and I think I inherited my uncle Wilbert's walrus moustache.* Seriously, wouldn't it be liberating? Think of the time you could save if you weren't constantly mowing the meadow. Think of a life without the pain of yanking every hair follicle on your body.

We buy countless products for our face. Lashes must look longer, eyes bigger, noses thinner, lips fuller, and our chins softer. I see an unhealthy pattern here. Young women never appreciate their unlined skin and taut bodies until they start to wrinkle and sag. Only then does an unlined face and firm skin become imperative.

Let us not forget thighs that resemble oranges, when pinched. Do yourself a favour, don't pinch your thighs. Moreover, under no circumstances should you place a pencil under buttocks or breasts to see if it will fall. It invariably will. If not today, tomorrow. Does the harsh clink of a pencil hitting tile diminish who you are? Is that all it takes for you to think less of yourself? It's rather sad and stupid if you give it some thought.

I could go on and on about how women are dissatisfied with every part of their body. Yes every part, think Brazilian, vajazzing (applying crystals or other adornments to your vagina.) Isn't it pretty enough? In addition to the latest trend: vatooing, that's right, tattooing your cha cha.

Studies have shown men look at their reflection and generally like what they see. We will not be their equal until we can look in the mirror and observe cottage cheese legs, junk in the trunk, and lined skin and still think we're desirable. If men can look past beer guts, hairy backs, and bald heads, we should display equal acceptance of our bodies. Men don't have to put women down, because we do a fine job of diminishing ourselves.

Connie makes her way to the waiting room. I follow her.

Radiation turns my right breast a nice bronzy colour. It no longer matches my pearly white left breast. That's what makes me think of the silly article. My surgeon removed four ounces of breast tissue. Before radiation, it's obvious my breasts are not the same size. Cleavage takes on a different meaning. Splitting divides the have from the have not. One cup runneth over, while the other doesn't come close to filling the chalice. As I near the end of my radiation treatment, my breasts don't match in colour, yet they look similar in size. Shading does make your boobs look bigger. Illusions aside, I face a problem. I can no longer wear clothing with an obvious centre. The cute little bow on my nightgown, or the straight seam on various sweaters, now skews to the right. I don't look up articles on the problem. I fear a staple gun will be involved. I understand why a lumpectomy at the twelve o'clock position is the worst location. It's the most visible. Pads can't fill out the missing plumpness.

I break the silence when I lean into Connie and remark: "You must be happy your treatment is over?"

"It's not over. I still have to do my boost."

"External beam?"

"Yep."

"It's only five treatments. That's not so bad. You're lucky. When mine is over I have to do brachytherapy."

"I wish I did."

"Why? External beam isn't as invasive."

I can't imagine someone wanting brachytherapy.

"Perhaps, but it doesn't go as deep. You're fortunate to have Doctor Stewart. He goes after that cancer with everything he's got."

"I'm sure the external beam is the best course of action for your particular case."

Her face bunches into a look of consternation. "Maybe, maybe not."

"What do you mean?"

Connie begins to frown. This time it has nothing to do with the outwardly changes that have taken place. "I think the cancer came back."

"Why would you think that?"

"I had a headache last night."

"So? You've probably had lots of headaches. It doesn't mean the cancer has travelled to your brain."

"My back was sore."

"Connie, you can't worry about it coming back. You haven't even finished your treatment. I'm sure you'll be fine."

"You don't know for certain," she says, huffing. She appears angry at me, but I suspect cancer is the offender.

"Do you really believe cancer is in your brain and travelling down your spine? Come on, you're going to drive yourself crazy if you blame cancer for every pain you feel."

"I'm already crazy."

Fear fires her eyes. The flame blazes wildly. Her tight body looks ready to crack. Cancer stole a year of her life. It appears she's willing to give it the rest.

"You have to have a positive attitude."

"Easier said than done."

"Okay then, if you can't be positive, be positively angry. Tell the cancer to fuck off. You're the boss. Tell it you don't want to see it again."

"I don't know if I can do that."

"Can't you at least give it a try?"

"I guess."

She begins to finger her wig. A moment later, she takes out her compact and checks her reflection. I suddenly understand. The complaints she voices is not what troubles her.

When cancer victims grumble about hair loss, water retention, thickening of skin, and so many other side effects, people say, or just think: *At least your life was saved.* That's what's important. They assume you should be grateful. They fail to understand how cancer stole the faith you have in your body. Trust is paramount regardless if it's between friends, or lovers, or between mind and body. Some fret about visible scars. Yet it's the fear they have in their body that tarnishes the image of themselves. Deceptive bodies appear ugly and threatening. They failed us once. They could do it again. The nastiest wounds are deep and invisible. Each of us learned a terrible lesson. What lies below may not be evident on the surface.

Prognosis aside, the fear of recurrence asserts itself. So is the knowledge that next time you may not be the victor. It's an unspeakable thought. You turn away from such a notion, pull out your compact, and check that your external self is in place. Better to do that than glimpse at the turbulence that lies beneath.

Cut, cooked and soon to be kaboobed, I joke about feeling like a piece of meat. I tell myself the incision on my breast has healed nicely. The one under my armpit didn't heal as well, but I decide it's easy to overlook. It's hiding in a crease. My two-toned breasts don't trouble me. The radiation tan will surely fade. As for the dejected wonky nipple, in time it'll perk up.

I nurse my hot breast with the flesh from the aloe plant I keep in the refrigerator, every day. Every night I use calendula cream, so not to burn and peel. I tell myself none of this bothers me. Am I lying? Unquestionably, but my intentions are good. I don't worry about a recurrence of cancer because I can't. I refuse to have worry as a constant companion. I don't want to peer over my shoulder, in fear of cancer catching me again. Am I brave not to face the possibility of a reoccurrence? Smart or stupid? Unsure of the answer, I do know it's something I don't want to explore. It's my life. Cancer will have the smallest fraction possible. If it catches up to me again, I'll deal with it, but I will not go looking for it. I will not invite it to share my life with me. I pray it won't be present at my deathbed.

*D*ARCY IS SITTING beside the aquarium, staring blankly at the colourful fish as they glide by. She looks unhappy; actually crabby is a better word. Her mouth, naturally wide and full, is a tight harsh line. Her blue eyes snap. She doesn't say hello when I enter the room. I vacillate over where to sit. I always sit beside her but I'm somewhat afraid to approach her. Irritation oozes out of her pores. Her clutched fists look ready for a fight.

I force myself to sit beside her. I try to think of something to say. "Nice warm day," I remark.

"Warm yes; nice, I don't think so. Look at my pants," she says, as she peers at the three-inch soggy band at the bottom. Salt stains are beginning to form and she scrapes at them with her pink fingernail. "I hate it when the temperature rises in the winter. It just makes a mess. All that slush ... Then the next thing you know it freezes over and you can barely walk without turning your ankle. And the traffic, it'll slow to a crawl. That is until the salt trucks are out and then everything becomes stained with salt. You think that's nice?"

I feel my chin jut out. "Yes, I think it very nice to walk down the street and feel a warm breeze on your cheeks."

Darcy's face bloats with displeasure. "You would."

"What's that suppose to mean?"

"You always see the cup as half full, don't you?"

"I don't see the point in making things worse." Getting up early, battling traffic and listening to a shrew is not my idea of a good start to the day. I might not have said anything, if she weren't glaring at me. "You're in quite the mood, aren't you?"

"What if I am?" she says defiantly.

Before we can say anymore, a technician calls her name. I'm happy to see her go.

I'm relieved when I don't bump into her in the hall. Before hopping on the table, I take off my red suede boots. My white socks are pink — and soaking wet. I fear they smell.

Rising temperatures do make winter messy. Nonetheless, the balmy weather tells you spring is just around the corner. That makes it worth the bother.

I'm lucky. I don't need positioning. As the days go by, I learn how to pose myself. Within minutes, my appointment is over. I change and head to the elevator. Darcy appears beside me. I ignore her.

"Sorry," she says, once the elevator's doors traps us in the five foot enclosure.

I look up at her. "You were rather nasty,"

"I know. How about if I make it up by buying you a cup of coffee?"

"Hortons?"

"Sure."

My walk is bouncy as I make my way to the car. I like Darcy and I'm glad we made up. Our argument feels like a schoolgirl scrap. I'm happy to leave it behind me.

A ticket flutters on my windshield, ripping the smile from my face. The ass of my car is passing the line by mere inches. Technically, it's illegally parked.

I snatch the ticket. Seventy-five freaking dollars!!%$#@$%

I scrunch it, but I do put it in my purse. The city, so desperate for money, always prowls the hospital zone. I'll pay it once I get home. I hope my money chokes the grasping bastards.

Darcy sits near the window. Today she's wearing a floral sweater. Dainty pearls dangle from her ears. A purse hangs from the back of her chair. It has to be from the 1940's. It's black with scatterings of petit point embroidered red roses. I'm sure the matching mirror and comb are inside.

Two steaming mugs of coffee sit on the table. As I take off my coat, Darcy says: "Triple, triple right?"

"Oh you remembered."

She nods. "How's it doing?" I know she's referring to my breast.

"It's fine. The aloe and calendula seem to do the trick."

"Lucky you. I'm burnt all the way through to my back. My skin is blistering and wet."

Poor Darcy had a mastectomy. Her fair skin is sensitive. I suppose it has to do with being a red head. The burning of her back might have occurred because she has no breast to absorb the rays. (My theory, not a fact).

"I can't take it anymore," she says.

I assume she's still talking about her breast. I'm wrong.

Her fingers wrap into a tight knot. "Ever since being diagnosed with cancer," she says, "people treat me differently."

Our eyes meet, and I nod. "They act as if you'll crack if they raise their voice at you."

"Exactly," she says. "They're killing me with kindness."

"Yeah," I say. "I especially hate it when they're annoyed with you. They're about to say something nasty, and boom, a look comes over their face, they smile, and say something entirely different. Luke does it to me all the time."

"Steve does it too. He's about to insult me, when he suddenly remembers I have cancer, and the next thing I know I'm being treated to dinner, or asked to watch my favourite movie."

"I guess they fear uttering unkind words," I say. "You may drop dead and the last thing you'll hear is — you're such a stupid bitch."

"If I am acting like a bitch, I would welcome hearing it," she says, pounding the table.

"But they can't say it. If they do and you drop dead, they'll surely go to hell."

"Steve's an atheist. So what's his excuse?"

"He'll go to hell too," I say. "The only difference is his hell will be of his own making."

Darcy's guffaw reverberates through the coffee shop. The three other customers turn to look at her. When it subsides she says: "Our families must think we're stupid."

"It's so transparent it's embarrassing."

"It's not natural. People don't act like that. It gives me the creeps."

"Censorship is never a good thing. I suspect a secret handbook is in circulation. Inside are ratings, similar to the ratings given to movies."

Darcy shrugs her wide shoulders. "You lost me."

"It's rather simple. A clandestine booklet. Unbeknownst to us, family members secretly get it after the diagnosis is made. Inside is detailed information on the etiquette on how to treat cancer patients.

As a cancer victim in stage one you would get a CVS1 rating, which means family and friends can still get angry at you, but must limit their retaliation to stern looks and puny words."

"Like don't be a silly billy," Darcy says with a snort.

"Yes, I think that would be appropriate for a CVS1. CVS2 would be gentle retorts like: It's that nasty treatment that's making my girl grumpy wumpy. Don't worry sweetie, we understand."

Darcy's eyes twinkle. She wears all moods blatantly. "What does my stage three get you?"

"A CVS3 rating gets you: Oh you're so cute when you're angry but all that cuteness must be making you sleepy. Perhaps you should take a nap."

"It must be said in a soft reassuring voice," Darcy adds.

"Goes without saying," I say. "And it's brilliant because they manage not to insult you, but nonetheless get rid of you for a few hours."

"Ingenious," Darcy says. "What's the rating for a stage 4 patient?"

"Stage 4 would get you a TFS4 rating. The proper protocol is adoring looks and soft words of love, regardless of what you're doing and what they really think of you."

"What does the TF stand for?"

"Totally fucked," I reply.

Darcy takes a sip of her coffee. "Maybe there is a handbook," she says.

"Maybe we should burn it," I suggest.

"Agreed, since it was obviously written by a moron and it deserves to be annihilated."

"I think the government is behind it."

"Probably. The material is worthless and, that's usually a sure sign of government intervention. If it cost a fortune to assemble, then we would know for sure."

We quietly sip our coffees. Darcy suddenly touches my hand. "You were right when you said I was in quite the mood. I snapped at you because this morning my husband ..."

I lean forward. "What did he do?"

Darcy's eyes look glassy. Tears wait for a blink to release them. Darcy doesn't blink. "My husband gave me a kiss after I threw an egg at him."

"You threw an egg at him? Was it raw or cooked?" For some rea-son I want to know.

"It was raw and I hit him right in the face. He had an important meeting scheduled so he was wearing his good suit and silk tie. The egg ran down his face, onto his tie and blazer and, when he bent to wipe it, it ran down his leg. One egg managed to cover him from head to toe and it wasn't even extra large."

"Thank God. You would have drowned him."

Darcy is sipping coffee. She unexpectedly joins me in laughter. It abruptly transforms to choking. Before I can become worried, coffee bubbles out of her nose. She froths like cappuccino.

That makes me laugh even harder. She frantically tries to get a ser-viette out of the dispenser but it's packed too tight. I'm now near hys-terics. I can't stop the snorting, and tears run from my eyes.

She gives up on the dispenser and reaches for my serviette. I pull it away. She suddenly growls: "Bitch."

"Gross pig," I retort.

"Skank," she counters, as she manages to pull out a wad of servi-ettes from the dispenser.

"Ass clown," I mutter as she wipes her face.

"Ass clown?" she repeats, somewhat perplexed.

"Do you like that one?"

"I'm not sure. Is it a real term?"

"It means that you are a skid mark in society's collective under-wear."

"I do like that. Do you mind if I use it."

"Feel free."

From that day forward, whenever we see each other, we mutter profanities. It makes us feel like our old selves and that's priceless.

*T*HERE'S A WOMAN I see every day. I never speak to her because she always has her nose in a book. The book acts as a barrier. It removes her from the circle of woman. After a few treatments, her nose withdraws from the book and faces a man called Daniel. He's also having radiation. For what form of cancer, I don't know.

I know the woman's name is Elizabeth because Daniel always calls out to her, and waves each morning when he enters the waiting room. Some days, I watch them. The attraction between them is obvious. They smile widely, laugh loudly and the room, crowded with patients, disease and caregivers, transforms into their private study.

Rings glitter on each of their fingers. They're married but not to each other.

Treatments progress. They sit closer to one another. I'm not normally nosy, but the situation intrigues me. Radiation will eventually end. Where will that leave them?

What good can come from a relationship that blossomed in such an environment? Am I going off in a tangent, created by my overdeveloped imagination? That one I can answer. No way. A brief look tells you they're wild for one another.

Days pass and I continue to watch their friendship develop. Given the circumstances it germinated in, I don't see how it can work. Having cancer myself, I can't see how nice people (yes I decide they are nice) can hurt their families, at a time when everyone is probably encircling them in love. I could never do it. It would spur guilt and guilt is one of the strongest fencing materials ever crafted.

I glance past my book and decide their attraction is still at the innocent stage. The closeness shared between lovers doesn't appear to be present. I wonder if it ever will be. Shared glances testify it could come to that. However, cancer is not sexy. It leaves you questioning if you will ever be desirable. The physical changes explain part of it. The psychological component holds the crux. When your turncoat body's treachery is exposed, you despise it. It's impossible to believe anyone can ever see beauty in it again. Maybe their libidos are not involved. If they are, I suspect they are hesitant and afraid.

When I'm sensible, I decide they're fools if they try to bring whatever they have into the outside world. It can never survive. When I'm romantic, I think to hell with caution, let the wind take you where it may. Cancer taught me the greatest measure of success is happiness. Unfortunately, it never revealed the price one should be willing to pay. When one grabs hold of happiness, he or she often yanks it out of another's hands. Is that a fact? Or unadulterated selfishness? Cancer never did say.

*C*AITLIN'S SHOWER IS today. Pretty boxes in shades of blue litter the house. It's common knowledge she's having a boy. I'm a horrible wrapper so I buy the nicest of paper, the biggest bow I can fit on the box, and yards of ribbon to cover corners that never manage to meet.

The shower is taking place at Heather's home, Caitlin's aunt on her mother's side. I have to drive my daughter, my mother-in-law, and myself across town, and be there by two o'clock. The day is cold, but dry and sunny, so I don't foresee any problems. We're all looking forward to the event, especially Madison.

"I can't wait for Caitlin to open my gift," she says.

This is the first time she bought something for a baby and it excites her. She coos over the tiny running shoes she purchased. It astounds me how everyone hates adult feet, but loves baby's feet. (Let's not think of fetishes). The tiny toes and thumb-sized foot is adored, even though flannel one-piece sleepers make them lethal. It is typical to see someone kiss a baby's foot, or put it in their mouth and pretend to eat it. I think it's one of life's odd mysteries.

My mother-in-law is in high spirits. "I bet Heather will do a good job. She loves to cook."

Checking the clock, I see it's one-thirty. "Time to go," I say, as I try to corral them out the door. My mother-in-law and daughter tend to be pokey. I'm not surprised when one has to go to the bathroom, and the other decides she needs a sweater.

It takes ten minutes to reach the car. As we head down the highway, I chat and pretend nothing is happening, but tamoxifen, my dear friend, is making the journey impossible. The side effect of the drug is hot flashes. In my case, it means a hot head that drips buckets of sweat and steams windows. The sticky vapour renders the wearing of glasses, sunglasses included, impossible.

Tamoxifen doesn't nudge you gently into menopause. It hurls you. The experience is akin to landing in Death Valley. Since conception, I've been cold. Suddenly I'm a human furnace. If you want to save on an energy bill, rent a menopausal woman. Turn down the furnace. Her body heat will keep the house toasty. She's also easy to annoy. Say something rude and she'll circulate the air as an added bonus. Some models attack housekeeping chores when provoked. It's a green solution. I wonder why no one has tapped into it? Or perhaps they have. Men may not be as dim-witted as we women like to believe them to be.

Why does he say such stupid things? He knows I'll get angry, yet he persists.

It's something to ponder ...

Driving one hundred kilometres, with the sun directly in my eyes, and unable to keep my glasses from fogging, I deliberate over how to prevent the three of us from dying on the highway. When I'm in the throes of a hot flash, I typically employ visual imagery. I imagine myself gliding down a frozen slide that encases me in a cylinder of ice. When I reach the end of the slide, I plunge into frigid water. I typically add a few penguins, and cute baby polar bears, to the scene. I usually shiver and glance at the animals before I return to the real world. Closing my eyes and visualizing frozen tundra doesn't seem like a good idea. I keep my eyes on the road and hope it will be over soon.

Every time I open the window to cool down, and rid the windows, and my sunglasses, of the slick moist film I created, my mother-in-law shivers. She is, after all, eighty-five. Cold drafts are not good for her, but I have to think of the common good. Driving blindly on a highway isn't beneficial to anyone's health either.

After I open the window for what must be a tenth time, Madison pipes: "Mom, don't keep opening the window. We're getting cold."

I ignore her.

When we pull up in front of Heather's home, my hair is curly and mascara streams down my face.

As she leaves the car, Madison remarks: "It's still winter, you know."

Not in my steamy world, where being hot isn't a compliment.

Heather greets us with a smile as she opens the door. Tastefully decorated, and festive, her home is inviting, as is the chatter of voices filling the rooms. I see Caitlin right away. She's eight months pregnant and oozes good health and happiness. Friends and family gather around her. With typical questions:

Is the nursery done?

Did you paint it blue?

Have you chosen a name?

"Yes the nursery's done. We chose yellow, in case our second child is a girl. We'll call him Nathan. No, not Nathaniel. Nathan."

We chat and play games. "Let's guess the circumference of Caitlin's belly," a young woman suggests.

Caitlin's face blanches. A good sport, she laughs when everyone guesses. She nearly faints when the measuring tape circles her waist. Her little fellow is taking up a lot of room.

When the platters of food come out, everyone digs in. It's as good as my mother-in-law thought it would be. I'm pleased to see the avocado dip, sitting in its heated pot. Prosciutto rolls around asparagus spears. Slivers of smoked salmon clutch cream cheese seasoned with onion. Shrimp peek out of pastry, as dollops of hot chili sauce dot their backs. Chocolate wafers look enticing as they innocently sit beside raspberries, swimming in syrup, accompanied by whipped cream. The large plate seems small, as guests sample a little of everything.

I enjoy the feast. "Coffee, tea and cake will be served shortly," Heather says, as I lumber around the room.

I love cake but I can't eat any more. A tea will suffice. A friend of Amy's, my sister-in-law, walks over to me. We chat about our children, who are similar in age. Suddenly she confides: "My mother had breast cancer."

I've known Lynn for years. I never heard of her mother being sick.

"Is she alright now?" I ask.

"Yes it was nearly ten years ago. It was a scary time." Lynn touches my arm. "But she got over it. Life returned to normal. She still goes for a mammogram every year and so do I."

Her comment makes me think of Madison. My breast cancer blemishes her genes. She's considered high risk. Breast cancer is the gift that keeps on giving.

I watch Caitlin open her presents, and wonder what the baby will look like. Will he resemble Caitlin or Kyle? What the child inherits is sometimes obvious, sometimes not. Madison inherits her looks from me. She has tiny features and looks young for her age. I hope she inherited my husband's health.

When it's time to leave, I give Madison the keys to the car. The sun is down. It will no longer blind me, but I don't want to be the driver. I covet the passenger's position. To sit, to think, to wonder ...

39

*S*ADLY, THE YOUNGER the woman, the more aggressive her cancer is likely to be. It's as if the cancer knows its prey is strong, and must calculate their strength into the equation.

My medical oncologist tells me the staging of cancer is not linear. "The difference between stage two and stage three doesn't change proportionally. In some ways, having stage one or two breast cancer is almost like having a different disease from stage three and four."

The stories I hear prove he doesn't overstate his summation.

I hear so many accounts of unbelievable tragedy, after awhile, I don't want to hear any more. A pregnant woman waits to start treatment until her second trimester. She wants to keep their baby. Beginning treatment during the first trimester can harm the foetus. Others give birth knowing their cancer is metastatic. Imagine giving birth, knowing you won't see the child grow up. I think of Caitlin and realise how lucky she is. She doesn't know it, because most of us can't imagine such a happy time in a woman's life being devastated by cancer.

When I'm filling out a questionnaire at the hospital, I hear of a girl, just twelve, diagnosed with breast cancer. They're scheduling her for a double mastectomy. Everyone talks about it in shocked tones.

How is such a thing possible? Breast cancer often remains undetected from anywhere from six to eight years. By the time you have the telltale lump, cancer has been squatting for some time.

Is the child's cancer so aggressive it grows at an alarming rate? Did it start when she was six?

She won't enter adolescence and see changes to her body. They'll take her budding breasts before they bloom. Will the doctors perform reconstructive surgery? How can you restore something that never was? Doctor Miller's words replay in my head: "I like to save breasts, because implants leave you without any sensations."

When my husband's aunt dies, people become evasive when I ask what killed her. It's my mother-in-law who finally tells me breast cancer took her life. "Ava's situation was totally different than your own," she immediately says.

"Oh."

"When she felt a bump, she ignored it. When she felt a second lump, she ignored that too. She turned away from her breast. Ava refused to see what was happening. She thought her blindness could change the situation. It did, but not in the way she wanted. By the time she saw a doctor, she was bloated like a balloon, and coughing endlessly. The cancer had spread to her liver and lungs. She was diagnosed stage four. There was never any talk of trying to cure her. The doctors only spoke of comfort and perhaps a few extra months. You went early. That makes it totally different."

I smile and say: "That's true." But I don't go to the woman's funeral. We are only so different.

Two weeks after the funeral, my sister-in-law, Amy, tells me her best friend's sister-in-law's breast cancer came back.

"She had a sore back and thought it was nothing. They were in Mexico, enjoying the sun. She waited until she returned home to check it out. She thought she pulled a muscle or something."

"How awful," I say.

"Yeah, everyone thought she'd beaten it. It was supposedly a closed chapter in her life."

That's how I see my cancer: A bump in the road.

"They told her the cancer spread," Amy says. "The diagnosis was bleak. She promised her husband she would beat it again." Amy's face falls, looking grim. "But this time it was bone cancer. I guess it's harder to beat bone cancer."

"Actually, it's still breast cancer. It has just travelled to a different location. That's what they mean when they say metastasis."

"I didn't know that. Anyway, that dream didn't last too long. Poor thing was in such pain, she was going out of her mind. The pain was unbearable. She had to go to the hospital and be drugged around the clock."

At this point, my stomach feels unsettled. "That's terrible."

"Yeah, it is. She wasn't very old. The same age as you, I think." Amy shakes her head. "Her husband can't believe he's widowed."

What! She died! I think my mouth fell open.

My uneasiness goes unseen. My sister-in-law continues with her story. "They had so many plans, so many dreams. The children are taking it hard. But near the end, everyone was praying for her to die. Her life became agonizing."

I'm shocked. I thought metastasis to the bone gives you years, not months to live. Her cancer must have spread to her organs and lungs too. I envision a wildfire running out of control, consuming the woman, as it ends dreams and severs relationships. This woman shared many similarities with me. I feel bad for her and her family, but selfishly I consider my family, myself. I don't want the story repeated, with my name injected into the narrative.

Amy starts chatting about something else. I pretend to follow her conversation. I nod and voice lame remarks. I think about what has taken place.

I don't want people to spare me, and censure stories. I'm not a child who needs sheltering from the truth. Yet, Amy's bluntness upset me. Cancer has changed me. I'm no longer the person I once was. Reality never frightened me before. People were never afraid to tell me anything. Insides were not something I worried about either. Metastatic disease and death were mere words. They didn't elicit a response. The person I allege to know inside and out is gone. My belief in who I once was proves to be an illusion. I never suspected cancer was growing in my breast. Proof of my ignorance pierced my potency and left me weak. You go about your life thinking, believing, everything is fine and then ... poof, the illusion shows itself for what it is. It transports you to an alternate reality, an accurate reality that doesn't consider your perceptions of what it should be. Are you a small part of that reality? No, you're not even that. You're insignificant. The realization chills.

I have become a stranger to myself. I have to get to know this new person. She seems flighty, unsure of what she wants out of life. Her inconsistencies baffle me. Does she seek coddling? Or does she stomp her feet and declare herself to be a strong able woman? She seems to do both.

The cancer is gone. The lessons are lasting. Will this tribulation strengthen, or weaken me? The choice is mine. I have power. Cancer's message can be positive or negative. So girlie, what are you going to do?

Who are you going to be? Do you want to be Little Miss Sunshine, or Doomschild?

Life is short. It doesn't come with any guarantees. I can worry about uncertainties or enjoy what life offers. I can be a victim of cancer or I can feel triumphant.

Some days it appears as if cancer is blowing in the wind and there's no escaping it. I can't outrun it. If it wants me, it'll find me. It has proven it can trespass into my body without my knowledge.

However, only I can allow it to encroach upon my mind. I refuse to give it admission. I will appreciate what I have. I will not wallow in fear. Life is fleeting. That's the key to its value. In the end, you have what you have and there's no point in asking for more. Shield your eyes. Here comes Little Miss Sunshine.

40

I'M HAPPY TO see Darcy sitting in the waiting room. Our appointments have not been coinciding. I miss talking to her. The other women are great, but Darcy and I are closer in age. We share more than just cancer. It also bothers me how the older women think I'm the lucky one.

"You're just young, not old like us," they often remark, as they cluster into a solid group. "It's easier for you."

I smile and never say anything when they make these declarations. But is it easier for me? Am I the lucky one?

My chances of reoccurrence are greater. Not trying to be insensitive, but if you are seventy-seven and were successfully treated for stage one or two breast cancer, it probably won't have enough time to come back and kill you.

Youth and cancer also have a turbulent relationship. I would never tell a thirty-year-old woman suffering from breast cancer that she's luckier than I am, because she's not. Her cancer is probably more aggressive than mine.

Finally, ignorance is bliss. Cancer's lessons are poignant, but I would prefer to live my life thinking I'm invincible. You're eventually proven wrong, but sometimes being wrong is preferable to being right. It's like an ugly person who thinks they're good looking. Their false perception makes them happy and confident. Why would anyone want to strip them of that?

Darcy sees me, smiles and pats the seat next to her. I hurry over.

"You wouldn't believe what happened," she says.

The news must be good. She's beaming.

She looks around the near empty waiting room. "Steve told me to fuck off," she says proudly.

I laugh and squeeze her arm. "Congrats. You lost your CVS3 rating."

"I did, but it wasn't easy. I had to nag him to near death. In his moment of weakness, I snagged that book of etiquette from his hands. Imagine treating me delicately! I ask you, do I look delicate?"

"You're many things, Darcy, but delicate isn't one of them."

"I know. Our marriage was never perfect. Few things in life are, but it was honest, and isn't that one of the most important aspects of a relationship?"

"Truth is very important."

"Losing that honesty was the worst consequence about being sick. When I found out I had cancer, my life began to spin out of control. I needed a constant. I needed something to hold onto. I needed our relationship to stay the same. Steve is the person I always count on. When he changed, I was devastated."

"Love ones focus on the physical changes, and overlook the need for stability. They see you as weak, and feel obligated to treat you gently."

Darcy plays with the chain of her satin purse. "Steve and I often shared gentle moments, but he never treated me as if I was fragile, at least he didn't before I had cancer. When he did, it appeared unnatural and forced. It was transparent. I could see his pity and fear, and I didn't appreciate it. Cancer weakens while treatment demands strength. I couldn't afford to have my strength questioned. My fortitude needed acknowledgment. What good is pity and fear? What does it get you? Holding back honest reactions doesn't help anyone; it only has the capacity to hurt."

Darcy continues talking. As the story unfolds, a satisfied smile replaces her annoyance.

"It took awhile, but he now knows that by treating me differently, I felt different. I explained what I needed the most was to be the Darcy I always was. I don't want illness to redefine me. I'm still strong and capable."

Her snappy eyes and fearsome stance make it easy to say: "I don't see how anyone can doubt that."

"Me either," Darcy says. "It was wonderful, Nan. We argued, we talked, and we made up, if you know what I mean?"

Her lewd look leaves no room for misinterpretation, but she pokes me in the ribs nonetheless.

"What about the kids?" Darcy has three boys and a girl. They too have been treating her with extra kindness. Does she want them to revert to what they were prior to her illness?

"Let's not get stupid. After working a full day, I can't go home, make dinner, and tidy up. As long as my relationship with Steve is back to normal, the kids can pamper me."

"Nancy Burns," the nurse calls. I get up and give Darcy's hand a squeeze before following the nurse.

I find myself in such an odd world. A woman beams because her husband told her to fuck off. Just goes to show you: honesty trumps politeness every time. I'm smiling as I make my way into the radiation room. I can imagine what Darcy did to extract such a retort. She must have made him livid.

"You're in a good mood," one of the technicians says.

"I guess I am," I say as I lie down on the cold steel table.

41

*C*AITLIN HAS THE baby. A boy, as expected. A huge boy, nearly ten pounds! She's in the same hospital I go to for my radiation treatments.

Poor Caitlin ends up having a caesarean. It leaves her exhausted. Luke and the children decide to let her rest for a few days, before visiting. They assume I'll go with them. I don't say anything but I can't envision myself going back to the hospital in the evening. I'm tired by the evening. Especially near the end of the week. The last place I want to go to is the hospital. However, I want to see Caitlin. I also want to see the baby. What to do, what to do?

Morning visits on the maternity ward are off limits. Time for the mothers to shower, rest, and spend time with baby and partner. I understand the logic. I respect the logic. I'll go as far as to say I agree with the logic. I'm also going to disregard the logic. Yeah, I think I'm special, outside the jurisdiction of rules. What are you going to do to me?

After I finish my treatment, I ponder how my niece and her baby are in the building next to me. I could walk there in under ten minutes. I don't want to bother Caitlin, but I do want to drop in and say hi. I want to see Nathan. I won't stay long. Just touch base, look at the baby, and then say goodbye.

I take a chance and walk over. If they send me away ... oh well, I'll drag myself back to the hospital with my family in the evening.

Getting into places I should not be in is one of my strong points. I act as if I belong. I walk with purpose. My stare is unwavering. My body language assured. It always works, unless I become lost and confused.

I can't find Caitlin's room. I begin to circle. My shoulders slump, my gait slows down. My eyes begin to dart.

Two nurses simultaneously pounce on me.

"Visiting hours begin at two," they bark in synchrony as they flank me.

"You shouldn't be here," one of them says. "This is the time allotted for mothers and babies, not visitors." She spits out the word, as if it's an offence to be a visitor.

"You have to leave," the other adds. They circle me like guard dogs. I hedge away from them, but they move in closer with every step I take.

With the weakest voice I can muster, I say: "Sorry, I didn't realize. I just finished my treatment at the cancer clinic. I was hoping to see my niece and her newborn baby. I'll try to come back during visiting hours."

That's right. I played my ace in the hole. The cancer card. Their demeanour instantly changes. They've been mean to a cancer patient. Oh no, what will happen to them now? I'm sure the etiquette book has a special chapter on offences and punishment for nurses. Their blunder will be seen as doubly bad. Both nurses look down at me. I look up at them and wonder what they'll do next.

"I wouldn't ask you to come back this evening," the chubbier one says. "It'll be too much for you. I'm sure your niece will be thrilled to see you." Then, suddenly cheerful and friendly: "Who is it you want to see?"

"Caitlin Bancroff."

"Room 304A," she says, as she points. Changing her mind, she grabs hold of my arm, ever so gently. "Let me bring you there." Once she deposits me at the door, she smiles.

"I won't stay long," I say.

"Stay as long as you want to."

Before letting go of my arm, she gives it an encouraging squeeze.

Caitlin is not alone. Kyle is with her.

"How in the world did you get in?" Caitlin asks.

"There has to be some benefit to cancer," I say.

My comical story makes it sound as if I accomplished a coup d'état. I don't validate the nurses' pity aloud.

I beam at Caitlin because I'm happy to see her. I hide my concern, underneath the smile. I see pain and weariness in her darkly circled eyes. Her movements are jerky. Her slim limbs are bloated. Her feet are misshapen. Kyle is smiling, but his body looks as limp as a wrung out rag. He hasn't left her side since she began labour. He sleeps on a tiny cot, alongside her hospital bed. Given his height, it has to be uncomfortable. Caitlin's story tells me their happiness was marred by the experience. I too had difficulty birthing. The agony abates when they place the child in your arms. The memory grows fainter every time you look into your child's eyes. Within a year, you're ready for another. I don't tell Caitlin this, because I think she'll kill me.

Kyle picks the baby up and offers him to me. I can't take him. Radiation is not supposed to adhere to me, and be detrimental to others. But I can't touch Nathan. He's too small, too vulnerable. Cancer and radiation should not be in his personal space. I tell his parents he's beautiful, and I mean it.

"Before I leave there's something important I have to tell you," I say.

Caitlin's face shows concern. I guess a cancer patient shouldn't use such an opening. I touch her hand. "I'm sorry to say this but you must buy granny underwear. Buy the ones that nearly touch your bra. I've had a caesarean. Bikini underwear line up perfectly with the tender scar. Your incision doesn't need elastic chafing it."

Caitlin and Kyle exchange a look. This is Caitlin's debut as a patient. She assumed the role would be fleeting. Her c-section and Nathan's jaundice augment the stay. Caitlin has learned one of life's dirty secrets. You can't count on life adhering to your schedule. Caitlin and Nathan will remain in the hospital for five days.

I only stay half an hour. Caitlin needs rest. I hand her a bag of her favourite jujubes. "For you, since you've done good."

As I walk down the corridor, back to the Cancer Clinic, I don't notice the blue dots. Instead, I think of the young family with so much left to experience. I smile.

*S*HE'S NOT A woman you can ignore. Her dark hair stands apart from the honey coloured sea of wigs. Her piercing black eyes exact attention. The air surrounding her appears frantic. She's only two or three inches taller than I am, yet she looms over me. The first time our eyes meet, she demands to know what form of cancer I'm suffering from.

"Breast cancer," I reply.

She's not wearing a double gown. Radiation isn't touching her breasts with its hot breath. Her presence makes me feel docile. Passivity feels unfamiliar and ill fitting. People usually don't overwhelm me, especially so rapidly and readily. I didn't ask her what form of cancer she has, but she tells me nevertheless.

"Do you remember Terry Fox?" she asks.

"Of course," I reply.

"I have the same kind of cancer: osteosarcoma."

No need to ask where the cancer is located. She's thin and wears skinny jeans. I can see swelling at the top of her leg. Unconsciously, her hand begins to rub the protuberance.

"Cancer is caused by the chemicals they put in water," she says, sitting next to me. "We're ingesting poison. That's why cancer is so prevalent."

I don't disagree with her. Manufacturers often have a blasé attitude when they use additives. Suffering, rather than research, has often fingered causal relationships.

We digress from like-mindedness when she blurts: "My doctors are furious with me. They want me to have chemo. They want to amputate my leg. They want me to have radiation. I have three of them badgering me, giving their opinions, and dismissing my thoughts." Her arms wave grandly. Her voice is fever-pitched. The other women look at us. She doesn't appear to notice. "They try to frighten me. Say I will die if I refuse all their treatments." Her arms fold across her chest. "They don't scare me. I only agreed to the radiation." Her face is defiant; her stance, aggressive.

She sees herself as strong and fearless. I suspect she's scared and unable to face reality. I don't tell her this. Instead, I say: "I hear chemo is tough, but it seems to be one of the best treatments for aggressive cancers."

"Chemotherapy is poison," she hisses through tight lips.

She digs in her purse, then hands me a pamphlet for a water filtering system. "I installed one last week. My water tastes better and the swelling in my leg has gone down. You must buy one."

I look at her and shrug.

Her eyes darken. "Do you want your cancer to come back?"

She glares at me, forcing a reply.

"Of course I don't want a reoccurrence."

"Then buy the filtration system," she says, as if issuing an order.

Before she can say more, the technician calls my name. I jump from the seat and begin walking so quickly the technician hurries to keep up. I'm happy to get away from the woman. She bothers me. I'm not fond of bossy individuals, but there's more to it than that. I'm just not sure what it is.

Darkness settles, radiation begins. I think of the woman. She provides cancer with a home. She dismisses caretakers, restrictions, and allows cancer to grow. Surgery treats cancer. Cutting off a leg is horrific but dying of cancer is worse. How can she dismiss the opinions of all her doctors? I don't believe in meekly agreeing to everything. If you disagree, say so, talk about, be convinced, or not, but be rational. If everyone is telling you that you're wrong, how can you not listen?

The next week I see the same woman talking to other patients. She speaks with the authority of a lecturer at a podium. I sit as far away from her as I can. I overhear her denouncing sugar. "If you withdraw sugar from your diet, you'll starve the cancer," she proclaims. "I already feel better."

My eyes meet Brenda's glance. She's a nurse I have come to know and like. Brenda remains quiet. She sadly shakes her head. She calls the woman's name. Sylvie leaves the podium after a second of hesitation. As she walks down the hall, I notice her limp. It is more pronounced than the week before.

I now know why the woman bothers me. I feel the fear in her screams. I see death in her emaciated face.

*S*WEAT DRIPS DOWN my face. I'm fully awake. I can still envision the dark-eyed woman who struggles with her doctors' counsel. She's little more than a stranger, yet she barges into my dreams as effortlessly as she barges into my waking hours.

I remember little of the dream. Yet remnants of fear cling to me. The overbearing, frenetic air of the woman still surrounds me.

She upsets me. Her fortitude is twisted and skewed, unknowingly angled towards self-destruction. Our interaction was brief. Nonetheless, I glimpsed the fear that blankets her, and obscures logic. She gazes sideways, as cancer attacks frontally. She dusts furniture during an earthquake. When a tsunami hits, you should not worry about water filters.

Her strength isn't helping her overcome obstacles. Instead of abetting, it disables. Her power mimics cancer. It rules in a chaotic manner. It plucks ideas and weaves them into a fabric that has no commonality to reality.

I suspect fear to be the foundation of chaos. Fear causes you to fly in every direction, without purpose. She must reorganize her power and face facts. Her convictions, her will, her dreams, none will conquer the cancer in her body.

I get out of bed. Grab a pen and paper. I often write when something inside of me needs to be dislodged.

Dear ...

As I begin to write a letter to her, I realize I don't remember her name. Suzanne, Sylvie? It doesn't matter. This stranger didn't touch me. She pushed. I skip the salutation.

> *I don't know your loved ones. I'm ignorant on how you interact with them. I presume you bulldoze their ideas, until the ground is flat, and only your thoughts flourish. They, loving you, respecting you, pitying you, say nothing.*

I do not love, respect, or pity you. I can speak the truth. The men and women who have spent decades fighting cancer are not your enemies. They may inflict pain, but their aim is not to hurt you. Think of the greater good. Use your strength productively. Battle through chemotherapy. Wear your wig with honour. When your body weakens, use your strength and spirit to force your damaged body to outlive the cancer that grows within you.

Prove to yourself and everyone else the loss of a limb em-powers in other ways. With every loss comes a gain. Use your courage to find out what yours will be.

Fight to live. Face facts. Battles may be lost, but the war can be won.

Do not confuse stubbornness with strength. Doing what you don't want to do takes the greatest courage of all. Open your eyes. See the true picture. You are going to die unless you do something. Don't listen to charlatans. Throughout history, the unscrupulous are always there to take advantage of the des-perate. They tell you what you want to hear. If you could beat cancer by taking a pill, filtering water, and reducing sugar, everyone would do it. Surgery, chemotherapy, and radiation wouldn't make sense. We would all use the magical pill and fil-ter our water.

Don't fall victim. You have the strength to be a victor. Follow your destiny. Be triumphant.

Cancer is a time in your life when a little selfishness is al-lowed. Take naps, long walks, watch your favourite movies. Pour so much bubble bath in the water that you are sheathed in glittering orbs. But remember, even cancer doesn't give you a ticket to ignore other people and their feelings and viewpoints. Allow others to touch you. Their arms reach out, not to take, but to give. They will strengthen you.

I reread the letter — and throw it in the garbage. It's not my place to tell her how to think. I wrote it to put my thoughts in order. The woman is a stranger to me, but the fear that radiates out of her every pore is no stranger. Cancer is scary. Cancer is chaos. Cancer can make the sane do insane things. Cancer makes you want to scream. I see no harm in screaming, but after you do, walk through the doors of the treatment centre and do what you must. I don't intend to organize someone else's life. Nonetheless, I wish her well.

Would I take my own advice, if our situations were similar? I hope so, but I don't know for sure. I turn off the light, fall asleep, and dream no more.

$\mathcal{E}$GGS. I HAVE to have them every day. After radiation, I hurry home and make an egg salad sandwich, or an egg with an English muffin and ham. It's somewhat challenging with my gluten intolerance, and high cholesterol. I've gained unnecessary pounds, and I'm often nauseous. Curiosity makes me google radiation and eggs. Have others experienced my obsession with the common egg?

Most of the information is about the eggs in the ovaries, and the effect of radiation on fertility. It is not my egg of interest. One article states radiation patients need more protein. That would explain my obsession. My body knows what it needs. I'm not going to worry about weight gain, and gastric problems.

I see Darcy in the waiting room and hurry over to her. "Do you crave eggs, since beginning radiation?"

Her face scrunches in disgust. "Are you kidding, I don't even want to eat."

"The opposite is true for me. I can't stop eating. It's starting to get embarrassing. My clothing appears to belong to someone else. I have a pre- and post-cancer wardrobe, ranging from size 4 to size 12. (Double digits, ouch)."

"I have noticed you've gained a few pounds, but I didn't want to say anything."

"You don't have to. It feels as if someone is following close behind, giving me wedgies."

"Buy bigger underwear."

"I refuse to buy size large underwear. Wedgies will be the punishment for my gluttony. They'll remind me to curb my appetite."

"I don't know if that's a good idea. You appear to be a slow learner."

They call Darcy's name.

I sit quietly, deciding if today is a sandwich or muffin day. Before I make up my mind, Francine walks into the room. She's older than I am, but young at heart. She tends to be chatty. I'm surprised when she doesn't sit beside me. Even more surprised when she doesn't try to start up a conversation.

I shrug my shoulders and look away, but my eyes keep going back to her. She looks different. Francine is tall and slim and usually well made up. Today she looks thrown together.

"How many treatments do you have left?" I ask, as I get up and sit down beside her. Normally I wouldn't impose myself, but her forlorn look tells me she's in need of a friend.

"I don't know," she says, in a lifeless voice.

Her answer doesn't make sense. Everyone counts down. Everyone knows exactly how many treatments are left. Like elementary school children, given gold stars for accomplishments, we know how many we're entitled to, and how many we already earned.

Francine's battle is similar to mine. She goes to her doctor, receives a clean bill of health, and four months later, while bathing, she feels a lump. She ends up having a lumpectomy and twenty-odd doses of external beam but no brachytherapy. She considers herself lucky. Until now.

"We just found out Bill has prostate cancer." She mutters the words so quietly, I lean into her.

Bill is her husband. When she started radiation, he accompanied her. Once she made friends, he came less often.

She's vague about how many treatments she has left because Bill shared breast cancer with her. He held her hand throughout the ordeal of surgery, and the seemingly never-ending rounds of radiation. They are embarking on a new journey of sickness. It's Francine's turn to hold his hand, and utter reassurances they both want to believe. She'll battle prostate cancer with him. She doesn't yet know his treatment plan.

It's not fair. She hasn't even finished her battle and she's about to begin another one. Cancer doesn't give a damn about fairness. It does what it wants for it has no conscience. It is Freud's id, without the ego or superego. Chaotic, it has no boundaries.

She looks at me and I don't know what to say.

"I'm so sorry to hear Bill is sick."

"They mentioned that treatment you were talking about."

"Brachytherapy?"

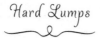
"Yeah, that's it. He doesn't want to do it."

"I don't either," I admit. It seems draconian, invasive, so ... intimidating. I'm thinking of telling my doctor I won't do it. I want my boost to be like everyone else's: five additional external beam treatments. I tell myself my reasoning is fact-based. Most of the literature on brachytherapy highlights the speed in which the therapy is preformed. It takes days, rather than weeks. Time is inconsequential, when it is only a boast.

I search the net looking for everything posted on brachytherapy. I'm surprised to learn some women opt to have their breast removed rather than spending weeks undergoing radiation. Brachytherapy solves that problem.

External beam radiation is a bother. No one wants to go to the hospital for twenty-three visits, but it's doable. I can't imagine cutting off my breast because I'm too busy. Who is that busy? I'm often in and out within a half an hour. Maybe the women who choose a mastectomy over external radiation live a great distance from the hospital. Perhaps they have no vehicle to drive to their appointments. Do some women fear dismissal because of the time required for radiation? The department opens early but, if you don't have a car, that doesn't help you. Luckily, an alternative treatment is offered.

Brachytherapy also emphasizes breast conservation. That benefit doesn't apply to me, since I'm not in the category of external beam, or brachytherapy. Instead, it's an addition. Radiation already affected my breast. I already spent my time. Five extra treatments seem preferable to having needles implanted in my chest. Who gives a damn if external beam takes three extra days?

Oddly enough my first reaction to Francine's admission is: "Maybe he should consider it. Brachytherapy works well on prostate cancer." Brachytherapy is a good choice, if you aren't the one who has to have it.

"I don't think Bill will change his mind." Her face looks grave. "He was rather adamant."

"Wait and see what happens. I'm sure he will get a choice of treatments."

"I hope so."

"Francine Leclaire," the technician says.

I watch them walk away. Francine was kicked in the stomach, once again. She didn't even have time to catch her breath.

I have to see my radiation oncologist, after my treatment. He sees me every Friday. He's always on time. Most visits are mundane.

"How are you feeling?"

"Fine."

"What about fatigue?"

"I go to bed a little earlier, but I can still do my daily tasks."

"How is your breast faring?"

"It's doing well." (It feels like a separate entity.)

"Is the skin peeling?"

"No, it's tanned but the skin is soft."

"Mind if I take a look?"

My answer is the raising of my sweater. During radiation, I don't wear a bra. The girls are happier unfettered.

"It looks good," he usually remarks. (At the end of the treatment, he congratulates it on doing exceptionally well. I feel as if someone I know received an award).

He makes notations. "What have you been putting on it?"

"Calendula nightly and I keep the pulp of peeled aloe leaves in the fridge. When I come home from my treatment, I apply it generously. It has a cooling effect but is gentler than an ice pack."

"You're not supposed to use an ice pack."

"I know. That's why I keep aloe in the fridge."

"It works well."

"Yes, it's cooling but not harsh."

My radiation oncologist is serious, meticulous, and hard working. A great doctor to have, but as people we have little in common. A personality profile would probably set us as polar opposites in most traits. It's not a bad thing. Different personalities are better suited to specific professions.

I'm nearly done with external beam radiation. We must schedule brachytherapy. It's time to broach what's on my mind.

"I don't want to have brachytherapy," I announce.

"I think that's a mistake," he says.

"After careful deliberation, I've decided against it."

He looks at me directly. His voice never changes in pitch. "Do you mind if I ask why?"

I don't want five needles, a misnomer if I ever heard of one; skewers would be more precise, thrust into my itsy bitsy boob. It's fucking gross and sounds like a torture treatment rather than a therapy.

Imagine going home with those things! How can you live with them for two days? What about sleep?

He suggests the treatment from the comfort of his armchair. Would he want the experience? They pierce through testicles as easily as breast tissue.

I just told Francine brachytherapy is effective in treating prostate cancer. I'm no different from the doctor sitting across from me.

There is one more thing about the treatment that upsets me. A private American clinic specializing in brachytherapy runs a horrendous ad. A woman has a lumpectomy. She ends up losing her breast because external beam radiation ravishes it. Using fear as a motivator upsets me, especially when it's exaggerated. I haven't met one woman who had such adverse reactions to EBRT that she had to have a mastectomy. If brachytherapy is so damn good, why do they revert to such smarmy tactics?

I also don't like how studies "are being done" to prove brachytherapy is as effective as external beam. Presently the results aren't in. I want concrete facts stating it is superior, not a hypothesis.

I don't say any of this. Instead, I say: "There's no proof brachytherapy works better than external beam, is there? Although there are fewer mastectomies when you employ brachytherapy, the survival rate is no different. As for breast conservation and time savings, well it doesn't apply to me since I will have already had twenty-three external beam treatments."

"That's true but you must consider that brachytherapy is more concentrated. It's especially useful when the cancer is deep in the chest."

I roll my eyes. "I might not even have second foci. The sample might have folded."

"Are you willing to take that chance?"

"No. That's why I want a boost, but I prefer external beam."

"I'll give you what you want, but I insist you to take a few days to reconsider."

"Intuitively, I feel brachytherapy is the wrong choice."

I give the young doctor credit. He comes back with his own sixth sense. "My intuition tells me you should. You're a perfect candidate and, since you may have a cancer deeper in your chest, I'll feel better knowing we gave you the best treatment available. Brachytherapy will cut your reoccurrence rate down to a third."

I know the statistics game. He's not telling me anything concrete.

"A third of what?"

"Thirty percent without brachytherapy, ten with it."

There you have it. Ouch.

I never wear a watch, because I will forever check the time. I never use an alarm clock, because I will forever wait for it to ring. I don't weigh myself, because I obsess over every deviation. I avoid numbers. They become too important to me.

I mumble something about giving it more thought. He has inadvertently found my weakness. Given my character, it's not one most would unearth. I can't ignore numbers. Numbers are flat and unyielding. Unlike words, which you can mould, and play with.

Imagine an airy-fairy who easily becomes obsessed with figures. Mere numbers shouldn't ground a person who thrives on chaos, and spends most of her time with her head in the clouds. It's an oxymoron. Damn him.

If I decline brachytherapy and the cancer comes back, I'll never forgive myself for refusing the recommended therapy. I've been through too much to allow that to be an option. I have no choice in the matter. I have to be kaboobed.

I could have told him he convinced me to go with brachytherapy. I don't. I suspect him of playing with words. Thirty percent sounds like the odds surgery affords without additional therapy. Did he consider tamoxifen, and the external beam radiation? I don't ask. I decide to make him wait. I didn't want to be convinced. I'm annoyed at him for doing it so effortlessly.

45

*J*HURRY TO the change room, ready to go home, when I hear what sounds like a snivel in the change room beside me. I ignore it. Not because my heart is cold but treading on someone's privacy is rude unless they invite you in.

As I leave the closet sized enclosure, I nearly bump into Elizabeth. She has nodded to me in the past, and I have smiled at her. But we've never spoken. It appears today will be no different. She seems distant, as if we're not sharing the same space. She stands in front of the lockers but makes no move to retrieve her coat. The change room next to me is now vacant.

My mother instilled politeness in me.

"Are you okay?"

"I don't think so."

"Is there anything I can do for you?"

"No, I don't think so," she says, ending our encounter succinctly.

I grab my coat. As I begin buttoning it, she asks: "Have you ever done something you know is morally right, but it feels wrong?"

What do you say to that? One can't answer this question without pondering: Had I? I can't remember. Perhaps I don't want to. She looks forlorn. I wish words would come to me. Not in the form of admissions, I won't give her those. But reassurances seem in order.

"I know I did the right thing, but I feel sick to my stomach."

Her dark brown hair appears black against her pasty skin. Her eyes look glassy. Elizabeth should be pretty. Her features are well proportioned. Her body is long and lean. Sadness surrounds her, distracting from her good looks. I touch her arm. I want her eyes to meet my own. "Would you like to get a coffee?" That's right, I ask someone who is nauseous to join me for coffee. I just don't know what else to do.

She hesitates. Then: "Yes that would be nice. That is, if you have the time."

I wonder what I've got myself into, but smile and say: "I have the time."

We go to a small cafe, a few blocks from the hospital. I drive us since she doesn't have a car. We barely speak during the ride. She sits beside me like a stiff overwrapped parcel. Coat buttoned to the neck, long, thick, scarf wrapped three times around her throat, and a woollen toque perched on her head. Overkill given the toasty temperature inside the car. Only when we slide into the red leather booth with our coffees does she loosen her clothing and speak.

"You had a lumpectomy, didn't you?"

"Yes, I did," I reply. "Did you?"

"Yes." She wraps her hands around her coffee cup. I fear we will resume our uncomfortable silence. Then suddenly: "Do you find it has changed how you feel about your body?"

I would normally say no. Something in her eyes makes me tell her the truth. "I'm self-conscious about it. Not when I'm in the hospital. The staff sees a lot worse. My surgeon did a wonderful job, but having breasts that are two different sizes and shapes and colours is not something I want. Variety might be the spice of life, but sometimes symmetry is the way to go."

She nods in agreement but doesn't add feelings of her own. "Do you still feel sexy?"

Elizabeth is an odd duck. She doesn't follow the protocol of acquaintances. I find her distant but, when she approaches, she zooms in much too close, leaping from silent to intrusive. Her forthright questions leave me resentful. She reveals nothing of herself, yet she demands personal information.

She leans into me and awaits my answer. I let her faux pas slide. She appears in need. When one is ill, it's a common practice to snare outsiders. Like weakened wild animals, you seize stragglers, because you don't have the strength to reach the centre. Outsiders are still nourishing. The sport is akin to psychotherapy, without the cost or commitment. I have the distinct feeling that, once we have this conversation, we will never see each other again. Elizabeth seems too confident for someone who has never bothered speaking to me before today. Courage habitually appears when there's no emotional involvement, and no chance of repercussions.

"I don't see myself as sexy, but I'm hoping to change my opinion," I disclose somewhat hesitantly.

"Do you see that as possible?"

If she didn't experience the same circumstances, her tone would insult. "Everything happened so quickly. It's difficult to keep up with the changes. I will eventually get used to them. I'm counting on the skin tone to return to normal. On good days, I'm happy everything went so well. It could have been much worse. I should be grateful. On darker days, I can't muster grateful. I resent what I had to go through."

Elizabeth's face darkens. Her hands become fists. "Since the diagnosis, I hate my body."

Her words are harsh. I'm not thrilled with my body's weakness. It allowed cancer to take over. It should have defended itself. A patsy, it didn't even recognize the enemy. Cancer fooled it into thinking it was benign. If only they could affix something onto the cancer to make the body realize it is under attack. *Do something you stupid fool!* But do I hate my body?

"Hate is a strong word," I say. "I think disappointed would be more appropriate."

Her dark eyes became snappish. "Hate is not too strong. If anything, it's not strong enough. I'm beyond disappointed. I despise my body. It let me down and now it's ugly. The lumpectomy left a dent. My breasts don't match and ..." She loses her words and does not continue.

"I'm sure it's not as bad as you think it is. You could have had a mastectomy."

"It wouldn't have been any worse," she says angrily, followed by a bitter laugh. "The physical changes are not what make me the angriest. The experience left me jaded. Too many people handled me. Touching me, seeing me, prodding me, was all in a day's work, and meant nothing to them. Yet in the end, I'm the one who feels like nothing. I detached myself from the situation. It made the encroachment bearable." Her hands unfold. "I can't find a way to reattach myself." She takes a sip of coffee. "You must think I'm crazy."

I find her atypical, but not crazy. "No, I know what you mean." I had never put her sentiments to words but, when she said them, I knew they were true. Every test, every exam, every meeting, is beneficial, but at one point the self is lost. You become a cancerous breast and little more. It's odd how touching typically leads to closeness, yet too much touching, by too many people, leads to detachment. "Time is a great healer," I offer, knowing the words are trite, even as they leave my mouth.

Her laugh sounds as brittle as her demeanour. "Perhaps you're right. I'm being silly and melodramatic."

Minutes pass. I dislike the truth she brings to the table. Suddenly she remarks: "I've noticed you watching me and Daniel."

My face surely reddens. It feels hot. "I couldn't help it," I say. "We were in the same room."

"I also think you know what happened."

"I have an idea but it might not be the right one."

"It is," she assures me. "I couldn't help it. The moment I saw him, I gravitated towards him. I don't know why."

"That sometimes happens." I gulp my coffee. Christ (Sorry God, I forgot), I don't know the woman. Why is she ending one awkward conversation, only to begin another?

"Not to me," Elizabeth says, playing with her wedding ring. "Today was his last treatment. He asked to see me outside of the hospital. I said no. He was confused. 'I thought you liked me as much as I like you,' he said."

"What did you say?"

"Nothing, nothing at all."

"Why didn't you say something?"

"I couldn't. I didn't want to admit how I felt out loud. When I didn't give any thought to what we shared, it seemed natural. But as soon as I thought about it, I realized it was inappropriate in too many ways."

She looks down at the table. She flicks a crumb. When she looks up, she's smiling, but it's a sad smile. "I don't want anyone to like me. I don't like myself. I can't handle affection. I can't understand it. It terrifies me."

"You're being hard on yourself."

She shrugs her thin shoulders. "That's how I feel. Cancer changed me. I'm not the person I once was. I'm not sure if I like this new person."

"It sounds as if you need to understand and accept your new self, before you can think about how others see you."

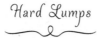
"It surprises me that he didn't see how damaged I was."

"You were scared."

"I was," she admits. Her hands flutter. "It doesn't matter; it's over now."

It was over before it even began, by the sounds of it. "Maybe it's for the best."

"You're probably right," she replies, but her words lack sincerity. She pays for the coffees and refuses my offer to drive her home.

I never asked about her husband or family. Now that she's gone, I wonder. Was her decision for the best?

He's a married man and she's a married woman. End of story. Succinct, but can a story conclude on one point? Are there other things to consider? Is her refusal to see Daniel for the best? When humans display their animalistic nature, they often find themselves caged and punished. The bars aren't made of steel, but they might as well be. We humans can coerce and confine with the power of our minds. We don't need outside forces to get the job done. Returning to the cage without being forced might be the best course of action. Nonetheless, she should have answered him. She should have been truthful.

I look through the window. Elizabeth is at the bus stop. Tightly wrapped, she seems oblivious to the cold. I think back on our conversation. Elizabeth's face was radiant and beautiful when she spoke of Daniel. A moment later, the bus arrives. She gets in. It's the last I ever see of her.

46

MY FRIDAY MEETING with Doctor Stewart arrives. "Fine I will do it," I say, even before my ass hits the hard chair. I'm finished arguing with him. He has won. He has the numbers and I, like a slave, have no choice but to blindly follow.

"You can do five external beam treatments instead," he says.

His expression tells me: both of us feel the last meeting didn't go well.

"I don't want to hear about options," I say. "Let's just do it."

"If you want external beam I can start working on the numbers."

He insists on giving me a choice, when it's no longer an option. His numbers frighten me. They scare away choices. Maybe it's a good thing. Maybe it's not. I'm not willing to find out who's right. I don't gamble. I'm not lucky.

I'm intuitive and imaginative. Often a perfect blend, but sometimes it's hard to separate what tool I'm employing. Brachytherapy provokes razor-sharp visual images. Am I feeding my trepidation with the revulsion of those images? Or is my intuition trying to warn me? I fear radiation can cause a different form of cancer. Submitting yourself to radiation therapy increases the risk of developing a second cancer, but only slightly. It also eliminates cancer. The benefits outweigh the risk of causing a second cancer later in life. Logically I shouldn't fear radiation. It's a friend, not a foe. Nonetheless, terror is present. The source is shadowy, beyond reach. Whatever the case, I made my decision. Sharpen the needles!

"After weighing my options, I've decided you're right. Brachytherapy is the best course of action. It can reach deeper recesses, and it causes less damage to healthy tissues."

Both statements are correct but my assertion is total bullshit. I'm not acting on rationale. I'm reacting to fear. The result is the same. The route is entirely different. Brachytherapy continues to elicit dark thoughts and terror. I don't embrace acceptance freely. When I think of it, my face scrunches up. Being forced to do something angers me. Defiant is a label often affixed to my chest. The fear of reoccurrence rips the label to shreds. Terror crumbles defiance easily. I toss my imagination and/or intuition out of the equation. I trust I won't regret the decision.

The young doctor looks at me and says: "I think you're making the right choice."

I smile and nod. I leave his office with an appointment set up with Doctor Martin, a specialist in brachytherapy.

47

SEVEN MONTHS AGO, I would've laughed in your face if you said I'd have five tattoos, own greasy camisoles, not wear perfume, or even deodorant, and flash my breasts to at least one stranger — if not two or three — a day. Body piercing to follow! Who knew I had it in me?

Doctor Stewart is not doing the implants. Doctor Martin is the specialist in brachytherapy. I'm supposedly lucky. He's one of the few doctors in the country who's qualified. I'm an ungrateful sod. I don't feel lucky.

I've never met the man. When I do, he immediately asks to see my breasts. It makes sense in my new world.

I lift my top and he grabs hold of my tiny Latina breast and squeezes. That's right my breast has changed. It's no longer the breast of a fifty-year-old Caucasian woman. It's small and firm, and feels prepubescent. I tell myself it makes me feel young. It's also a different colour from the rest of my skin. I christen it Niña Lola, which means little girl who is sorrowful. It makes me feel exotic. Prior to the lumpectomy, I had two small breasts. Since the surgery, I have a small, and a big breast. It almost makes it sound as if they gave me something, rather than taking something away.

Doctor Martin appears to be a happy man. He's always smiling. He also dresses well. The only doctor I saw who wears a suit and tie. "What do you know about brachytherapy?" he asks, after the squeeze and assessment. (I admit his smile makes him appear ghoulish. I was wrong about health care workers appearing sombre. At least some times. We could laugh and joke afterwards, but while he's talking about plunging needles into my chest, I want melancholy.)

"I know very little about brachytherapy. It must be something new."

"Actually, you couldn't be more wrong. It's one of the oldest radiation treatments. Brachytherapy treats the cancer from the inside out."

"So it immediately targets the problem."

"Exactly. It's highly effective and doctors have been using implants for over a hundred years. The first brachytherapy treatments began after Roentgen discovered X-rays, and Marie and Pierre Curie established radioisotope extraction."

"Wow that long ago. That's interesting."

"I think so.' He claps his hands. "Enough about history. Let's return to the present. I'll be inserting five needles, horizontally." He takes out a piece of paper, draws a breast and five needles protruding from it.

I find the visual so unnecessary.

"I always do the procedure early in the morning, so you can have your first treatment and arrive home by early afternoon. I want you to be at my office by seven-thirty."

"The earlier the better," I say with a gulp.

"You'll be awake during the surgery but the anaesthesiologist will give you something to block the pain, and also something to forget the experience. After the procedure is completed, you'll have one treatment, go home, come back to the hospital the following morning, have another treatment, go home, and return in the afternoon to have your final treatment. The needles will then be removed."

He smiles throughout his explanation. They'll erase my short-term memory! They'll plunge needles into my breast! It's chilling and I say so.

"Five needles running through my chest sounds invasive and frightening. Rather high on the yuck factor if you know what I mean."

"I do. Everyone feels queasy when I explain it to them. Even other doctors." He says this with a chuckle. "When I go to conventions, they tell me to put away the photographs. However, most women say that it's not as bad as they thought it would be."

Yeah, once it's over.

"It also has no side effects."

"A definite bonus."

"Within a few weeks most women look as they did prior to the procedure. It's very concentrated and doesn't damage healthy breast tissue. You need not worry about the effects it has on your heart and lungs."

"You mention treatments, but I don't really know what you mean."

"You're having HDR (high dose rate) brachytherapy. During your treatment, a radioactive source (radiated seeds) comes out of a machine called a high dose rate afterloader. The seeds travel through plastic tubing to the catheters in your chest. We do this under computer guidance. During your treatment, you'll be alone in the room. The radiation is left in place for only a few minutes at a time. Our focus is where the tumour was. It's an outpatient procedure which usually takes fifteen to twenty minutes."

I'm nodding dumbly. Perhaps I can get a job like those dogs people once had on their dashboard. My stupid, sappy, nodding intends to mask fear.

"Do you have any other questions?"

"No. I think I understand."

"Shall we book your appointment?"

"Yes please." (I'm so stupidly polite.)

"I'll get my nurse to call you with definite dates. Would you prefer the beginning of April or the end?"

"The beginning of April would be best."

He stands, shakes my hand, and gives me the diagram of the breast with needles running through it. "You'll get a call within a few days."

Ya, see you soon, Chuckles. When he leaves the room, I throw his drawing in the wastebasket. It disturbs Niña Lola.

48

*W*HEN I GO to the optometrist, I have the sudden urge to place my breast in the chin guard. I'm no better than Pavlov's dogs. Until that day, I didn't realize the extent of my training. My recent experiences tilted my world. My centre is my right breast. Odd, since after adolescence I gave little thought to either breast.

I'm making up for my neglect. Some days I must remind myself not every twinge and ache is related to my breasts and cancer. They're the bad days. I think of the advice I gave Connie, and tell the cancer to fuck off. Unlike her, I do angry very well.

My optometrist asks if I'm on any new medication.

"Tamoxifen."

She doesn't react, which tells me she doesn't know the usage of the drug. Cancer always gets a reaction. As the exam progresses, I find myself telling her about my fight with breast cancer. When I discuss the disease, it's often to acquaintances. I don't talk to those who are close to me, for fear of upsetting them. They don't talk to me about cancer, for fear of upsetting me. The circle of evasion is difficult to break.

My optometrist knows very little about breast cancer. She reminds me of myself prior to my diagnosis. Sure, we women all have breasts and we've all heard about breast cancer, but most of us give it little thought.

The first words out of her mouth are typical. "Did someone in your family have it?"

She seems taken aback when I say: "No."

No one likes to have a comforting blanket pulled from them. Every woman wants to hear how you were at greater risk of breast cancer than she is. A false sense of security is preferable to cold reality. Why be overshadowed by the threat of breast cancer, when no one in your family had it? Answer, you could be the first to walk out of the sunshine, into the gloom of malignancy.

I always tell women who are approximately my age that I didn't have any significant risks of developing breast cancer. Do I want to scare them? Yeah, I do. Consider it a warning, similar to: Do not walk alone in the park at night.

Common sense: it can happen to anyone. Time spent worrying is time wasted. Time spent having a yearly mammogram is time well spent. I don't want anyone to be like me. Only after a suspicious mammogram and a telltale ultrasound did the notion become clear. Anyone can have breast cancer. If I had realized that, I would not have dismissed my little lump so easily.

"You look so healthy, you look so young," she says in amazement.

That's the point I'm trying to get across. As the cancer grows in your body, you don't look sick. You don't even feel sick. As for age, there is no magic number. I had a little lump that didn't even appear to remain static; I didn't have any symptoms.

Before I leave, she admits to not having a mammogram in a long time. "You get so busy," she explains.

I look at the photograph she has of her four children and husband. "I was too busy too," I say with a smile.

I hope she books an appointment.

49

J'M FINISHED MY EBRT (external beam radiation therapy). I'm thrilled. My last gold star is in place. The magnificence of my stellar collage glows brilliantly. It's over! Eureka.

No more waking up early.

No more battling traffic.

No more searching for free parking.

No more strangers leaning over my half-naked body.

I wake up the following morning. I expect to feel overjoyed. I wait for it, but it never arrives. Instead, a feeling of being lost shows up.

Rushing to the hospital has become a routine. I wake up on schedule. I promptly forget the exasperation of battling traffic. The hassle of finding free parking doesn't seem so bad. I miss my morning walk. I miss talking to the other women, and the staff whom I genuinely like. Days pass. I understand why some women feel anxious instead of thankful when it's over.

Cessation of treatment severs your safety net. Unknowingly I became reliant. Sharing concerns with the other women gave me strength. Sharing divvied our qualms, leaving no one holding the full bag. Sharing validated thoughts, proving worries are a normal part of the healing process. The surgeon's scalpel doesn't cut all the cancer. Disease often remains in the form of malignant thoughts and irrational fear. Radiation doesn't eradicate doubts. You don't reach wellness in a single bound. You move away from cancer like everything else — one step at a time. Surrounded by women who struggle to reach a singular destination, a collective purpose that fortifies the mind and soul.

Throughout the process, constant tests infuriate, constant touching makes one's skin crawl but, when it's over, you yearn for the security of constant monitoring. Examinations terminate, while doubts begin. Is everything still okay? You tell yourself: everything is fine. However, your voice can't overpower the nattering that questions: *What about now? What about now?* Like a bratty child, the voice refuses to listen to reason.

I prize my independence. I always have. I'm shocked when I must relearn how to stand-alone.

Unfortunately, Jackie's mother makes me appreciate how lucky I am. She's still in the throes of cancer. She's awaiting surgery. Her chemotherapy — six treatments, at three-week intervals — extends the cancer experience. My surgery is a distant memory. My external beam radiation has ended. I still have brachytherapy ahead of me, but a two-week interval seems great, when one is accustomed to daily medical appointments.

Madison and Jackie communicate via text messages. Madison is upset when she reads the latest.

"Jackie's mom can't have the surgery yet. The tumours have not shrunk enough. She's scheduled to have three more rounds of chemotherapy."

I feel for the woman. I don't know her, but part of me feels as if I do. We share a common acquaintance. She knows him better than I do, but I know him well enough to know ... Life can be so difficult.

Madison doesn't have the particulars, but I'm sure Katherine must be stage three. I pray the additional rounds of chemo will shrink the tumours so she can turn her back on our grey weather friend and move on. Her troubles clarify, cut through petty concerns ... I must appreciate how my life is once again my own.

The additional chemo shrinks the tumours. Three months pass before Jackie's mother can have surgery.

Her options differ from mine. I chose between a mastectomy and a lumpectomy. She could have a single or double mastectomy. Large breasts convince her to have the double. A weakened body forces her to have a single mastectomy. She can't survive the trauma of the removal of both breasts. She has the single mastectomy, and her body slowly heals.

Her spirits, which were low through this whole ordeal, lift once surgery is over. Two Rottweilers sitting on her chest weighed her down.

She now wears a prosthesis. She'll wait a year, to give her body a chance to recuperate, before having another mastectomy and reconstruction. Next spring she'll have two new breasts. This spring she has one breast and the belief that a large part of her life is still before her. She and Jackie are planning a wedding. Jackie and Brendan will be married next summer.

*D*OCTOR MARTIN'S NURSE calls. She has a sweet cheerful voice. "There is an opening on April 1st at seven-thirty. Are you interested?"

April Fool's day. What a wonderful day to have surgery. Will I arrive to find out it's all been a hoax? Not likely. April 1st isn't a statutory holiday. Everyone is still at the grindstone. Some are sharpening needles.

"April 1st would work out well."

It's three days before Easter but I've already resigned myself to my cancer's obtrusive behaviour. It always wants centre stage on holidays. Its reign of terror will soon be over so let it have its last hoopla.

First century B.C. writer Publilius Syrus once said: *Formidable is that enemy that lies hid in a man's breast.* I take his words as wisdom. I'm grateful to have my enemy stabbed. The crossfire catches poor Niña Lola. I can do nothing to save her. She's like the idiot in a horror movie who walks down the darkened alley. *Don't go, don't go,* you mutter. They invariably make their way into the darkness. It's their destiny.

"We provide ginger ale but, if you want food, you'll have to bring it yourself," Nurse Brenda informs me.

"That's fine," I say. "How long will the procedure take?"

"About an hour and a half."

Ninety minutes to plunge five needles into my breast. Does that include marinating?

"Do you know where we're located?" Brenda asks.

"Aren't you at the Cancer Centre?"

"We are, but we're a little tricky to find. When you come to the clinic, take the elevator at the main entrance. Go to the second floor, but exit from the back of the elevator. If you don't, you won't be able to find us. When you get off the elevator, we're the first door on your left."

"Fine, I'll see you on Wednesday."

Wednesday arrives quickly. Luke accompanies me. He hates how I wrote the directions on a napkin, in a sloppy haphazard way. He's sure we won't be able to find the place.

My directions lead us to a frightening door. It has signs plastered all over it. *Do not enter. Danger, radioactive material.* My imagination adds skulls and crossbones. Apprehension paints the door a brilliant shade of red. My conception of the portal to hell. Internal alarms sound. The blood pulses through my body with a mighty clatter. I don't want to go in there.

My hand touches the knob.

"Don't touch it," Luke hisses.

He's sure we are at the wrong destination.

"Don't go in there," he whispers with the type of urgency I can only muster when I scream.

I ignore him and push through.

The door opens to a lacklustre waiting room. Typical and a tad ratty. A nurse with grey hair and a welcoming smile says: "You must be Nancy. I'm Brenda."

Brenda's appearance matches her voice. The laugh lines around her eyes and her quick smile speak of an even temperament. I attempt to smile and fail. Brenda must be accustomed to grimaces.

"The doctor isn't in yet. Take a seat. I'm sure he'll be here shortly."

We sit on worn pleather chairs. The portal opens with a squeal. Mrs. Adams enters.

Last time I saw her, we were parked in a hallway, awaiting surgery. The first words out of her mouth are: "You lied. The needle did hurt. It took five tries before they finally got it in."

It takes me a second to realize she's referring to the wire localization with the accompanying Dixie cup. I didn't lie. The technician got it in on the first try and she didn't hurt me. Five tries sounds excruciating but, considering our breasts are about to become tits on sticks, the localization seems trivial.

Prior to surgery, Mrs. Adams had two daughters at her side. Today only one remains. Her eldest lives in Calgary and couldn't make the trip down.

"You're preceding me again," she remarks.

"It looks that way."

"Don't bother telling me how it goes."

"I couldn't tell you even if I wanted to. My short-term memory will be wiped clean."

A moment passes before she asks: "How many needles are you getting?"

"Five, what about you?"

"I'm also getting five."

Brenda is puttering in the adjacent room. The noises she makes sound thunderous. I want to ask Mrs. Adams how she feels about the treatment, but with Brenda near-by, it doesn't seem polite. My viewpoint would include a litany of curse words. Instead, I ask: "Do you know anyone else who's getting brachytherapy?"

"No, only you."

"I guess we're the lucky two."

"Why are we getting it?" she asks. Her churlish tone tells me we're two ungrateful sods.

"Didn't you ask Doctor Stewart why he picked brachytherapy over an external beam boost?"

"No, of course not," she says indignantly. "He's the doctor and I'm the patient." Mrs. Adams doesn't lack the qualifications of a patient. Prim and proper, she can't bring herself to question her doctor.

"We talked about it," I say. "He said he wanted to radiate deep in the chest. Brachytherapy is precise so you needn't worry about inadvertently radiating the heart and lungs."

"He didn't tell me about that," she remarks through thin lips.

Doctors often take cues from their patients. If you don't ask questions, they don't volunteer information. Many of the women I meet don't understand even the basics of breast cancer. Quite a few don't even know the stage of their cancer. They dispense their disease to their doctor. *Here take it. Don't bother me with it. I'm not qualified to deal with it. I don't understand it. I don't want to understand it. I want my life back. Please give it back to me.*

It's akin to hiding in a bomb shelter while others fight the battle. Only when it's safe do they stick their head out. If the battle is lost, you have to drag them out of their sanctuary and force them to acknowledge defeat.

The door opens with force, and bangs against the wall. Doctor Martin zips through it, smile in place, paper coffee cup in hand. He keeps walking until he passes through double doors on the far wall. I assume that's the surgical area.

Brenda leads me to the change room, hands me two gowns. "You can retain all clothing below the waist, with the exception of your shoes." She hands me blue paper slippers, which match the gowns. They appear senseless. They slide on the tile floor, stealing my sure footedness. Their logic lies in diseases and foot funguses. If everyone walks bare footed, disease will spread. I agree but ... If I fall down with those skewers in my chest, I'll scream bloody murder and the situation will reverse. The portico to Hades will open, and swallow them in one vindictive snap.

Once dressed, I find myself on the surgical table. The anaesthesiologist stands above me. "Hello. I'm Doctor Sullivan."

"Hello," I croak. Witty repartee eludes me. Doctor Sullivan is wearing a mask. I only see his eyes.

"Don't worry about a thing. You'll be awake, but feel no pain. Once the surgery is complete, I'll give you something to block your memory so the experience will be hazy."

"Great," I mutter flippantly. "I don't want to remember any of it."

He takes my words at face value. The clanking of bed rails, clicking into place, is the first memory I have of the experience.

"I guess I fell asleep," I remark, to the blonde nurse who hovers above me.

"No you were awake the whole time," she says. "You've been talking to me for over an hour."

My trip is over. I disembark and find myself in the land of Alzheimer's patients. It feels lonely and frightening. I never saw that woman until a few seconds ago. I have no recollection of talking to her. I have the urge to lie.

"Oh yes, how silly of me. Of course I remember talking to you."

"You told me all of your dark secrets," she says, jokingly. Her smile is conspiratorial. We must have interacted. I have no idea what I said to her. The situation leaves me uncomfortable. I cover my vulnerability with a smile and a tinny giggle.

Brenda comes over to my bed and tucks in blankets. I'm then ginger ale'd. (Yes, it is a word, a medical treatment used for all afflictions.) She leaves the room, but I'm not alone. Curiosity keeps me company. We immediately get into an argument.

"Take a peek," it says.

"No, I shouldn't. It'll gross me out."

"Come on. Don't you want to see what they did to you?"

"It's not prudent."

"Prudent, shmudent, don't be such a baby. Have a look see."

I throw the covers off, lie perfectly still, and check that no one can see me. Assured that I'm out of everyone's line of vision, I pull the gown away from my chest, and peer down. Holy shit, I'm kaboobed. Five skewers run through my breast. Red rubber ends stop them from moving. Niña Lola is blackened and trampled. She could star in a horror movie.

Brenda returns. "Are you hungry?" she asks sweetly.

I'm not, but it's easier to say I am. She'll keep asking until I eat something. "I have mango slices in my bag. I wouldn't mind a few." Brenda gets them for me.

"I eat mangoes all the time," she says. "I never knew you could buy them dried."

"Try some," I say, holding the bag out. "They're very good and not messy."

She takes one slice. "It's delicious."

"Take a few more, I have plenty."

She smiles shyly and takes a few more. The forgettable blonde nurse moseys over. She peers at the bag.

"Try some," I encourage, as I take a few myself and sip on my ginger ale.

"You have a good appetite," the blonde nurse remarks.

"A little too good. I've gained at least twenty pounds since finding out about my cancer."

"Same thing happened to me," she says as she helps herself to a few more slices.

"When did you have breast cancer?"

"Two years ago, next month, and I never lost the weight I gained."

She's about my height. Our asses are similar in shape. Both are round and bubble like, rather than flat and wide. Her buttocks stretch out her white cotton pants. Her words annoy me. It's bad enough to have had cancer. It's not fair to be left lugging a fat ass around. After all the crap I've endured, I should at least be thin.

Squeaky wheels announce Mrs. Adams' arrival. Brenda parks her bed next to mine.

"Are you hungry?" she asks her.

"I am," Mrs. Adams says.

Seems Mrs. Adams didn't remember to bring herself food. I hand her the bag of mangoes.

Mrs. Adams is older than I am. Her personality is much more serious and calm. She appears to be a nice person, but I gravitate towards louder, funnier individuals. Life is too serious to take seriously.

Whatever our differences, fate insists on crossing our paths. We become grey day companions. We share surgery, and we share brachytherapy. We share feelings, thoughts, complaints, and our histories. She refused chemo because her husband was horribly ill during his treatments. Unfortunately, he died three years ago.

"I ended up getting seven needles," she remarks.

Why she's still calling them needles is beyond me. Come on, lady, look at them. Needles don't look like that. The catheters are as thick as pencils.

"Did you take a peek yet?" I ask.

I earn another pucker face. "No. And I don't intend to."

"Do you have any memory of the surgery?" I ask.

"Of course, I remember all of it."

I don't tell her I can't remember any of it. How much of the drug did Doctor Sullivan give me?

The clock strikes twelve. Brenda comes for me. She's smiling but it doesn't make me feel any better about my first treatment. She helps me out of bed and steers me into a wheelchair. I could easily have walked, but protocol is the big honcho in large institutions. She wheels me to the radiation department I know so well. I expect the elevator doors to open to the familiar waiting room. Only an empty carcass remains. Tables littered with free knitted caps, for baldheads that become cold at night, no longer hide in corners. The mammoth fish tank, a central attraction, is no more. Chairs don't jut out into parallel lines. Women's asses don't keep the seats warm. The front desk, which was always a bevy of activity, is strangely quiet. Only Suzanne, the receptionist, is there. "I haven't forgotten about your crown, princess," she calls out when she sees me.

I don't feel like a princess. The land I knew so well feels pillaged. The squeaking of the wheelchair echoes through the hallway.

Brenda leans over me. Her hair smells flowery. "The radiation department is moving."

"I wondered why it's so quiet."

"There are very few patients left. The new plan makes sense. Instead of seeing your doctor at campus A, having treatment at campus B and then having tests wherever, they're going to have everything at one centre."

"That does sound more efficient."

Nonetheless, I see a page of my history rip before my eyes. My right breast begins to throb.

As if reading my mind, Brenda asks: "Do you feel any discomfort?"

"I'm starting to feel a twinge."

"I'll give you some hydromorphone to keep the pain at bay. Do you have any left over from your surgery?"

"No," I say, lying. "The instructions said to throw away any unused medication so I did."

I actually used very few of the forty pills prescribed. I don't take drugs unless I have to. I understand addiction on a cognitive level, but I don't understand the pleasure one derives from drugs. They make me feel sluggish and often nauseous. My drugs frequently expire. Nonetheless, I keep them handy in case I really need them.

"I'll make sure you get another prescription," she says.

I wait for my pants to ignite. They don't.

I've always gone through the doors on the right hand side of the front desk for my external beam therapy. Today I'm going left. The room I enter is large and well lit. Boxes are perched in a corner, lying in wait, anticipating their involvement in the big move. The few things not boxed seem out of place, anxious.

I get out of the wheelchair and make my way to the table. My fear of touching the needles makes my step as unnatural as the Frankenstein monster's wooden gait. A petite blonde woman smiles at me. There are many blonde women working in hospitals. Like Hollywood starlets, I'm beginning to mix them up. As she helps me onto the table, we discuss our plans for Easter. She goes to the computer and feeds it relevant information. It makes happy, smacking sounds. We chat about ham and homemade pies. She removes the gown from my shoulders. My breasts remain covered. She discusses her guest list. She pushes the gown down. The mundane conversation mixes with the intrusive procedure and leaves me quiet.

She leaves the room to come back with a camera. Upon seeing it, my body tenses. "We take photographs to keep in our records," she explains. Her words are quick and logical. Click, the sound is harsh. Niña Lola is compliant as the technician takes her picture.

"Don't worry, it's not a headshot," she says as she carries the Polaroid away, without showing it to me. An image of participants at future conventions flashes in my mind. I envision the audience as it turns away in repulsion at the sight of poor Niña Lola.

They take without asking. Is permission mandatory only when your whole is violated? Pieces do not count. At what point do parts of your body become a human being? Can you feel human when dissected?

The red nibs pull off easily. The connection to the remote afterloader is made. Danger often wraps itself in darkness. Gaiety typically flourishes in brightness; however, the fluorescent lights that shine down on me feel cold. They pitch me into an alien environment. The cables connect to my catheters, as snakes fastened to prey. I yearn darkness. I don't want to see.

She's just about out the door when she turns to face me. "There are cameras in the room and an intercom. You can talk to me if you want to." Her words are an afterthought. I nod but wonder what one says in such a situation. Idle chitchat seems silly. Philosophy, politics, religion, all seem unsuitable. What would happen if I screamed? She would listen but surely she wouldn't enter the room until the procedure was complete. I don't blame her. Why should a healthy person risk radiation?

The computer knows I'm alone. It tells the afterloader which begins to spew radioactive seeds. They click sharply as they thrust towards the catheters in my breast.

PING, PING, PING.

They move closer. They hit their target and bustle back to the afterloader. No radioactive residue will remain once the treatment ends. Do the seeds pilfer anything as they dash away? The treatment only lasts minutes.

The blonde returns and we carry on our discussion as if there was never a fracture. She disconnects me from the afterloader. I'm free to go.

"I'll see you tomorrow morning at nine," she says, before I step into the hallway.

I ARRIVE HOME. It looks the same as it always does: books litter tabletops, cords from computers peek out from under couches, the smell of cooked apples fills the air. But the feeling of alienation rests in the skewers. They pierce the familiarity and leave me unsure of what to do with myself.

Should I ignore them? *What skewers? What are you talking about?* That would be full repression. Absolute denial. I could also employ partial repression. *My breast has always had horns sticking out of it. The alloy and rubber tips are natural. Of course, it doesn't hurt, but it does make air travel a bitch.*

Drawing attention to them is another option. *They stuck skewers through my breast! All I did was lie on a narrow table. Upon becoming cognizant, I found catheters protruding from my breast. Ten blackened puncture marks assure me it's not a nightmare. If only it was. For when I open my eyes, the abomination remains.* Or on a more succinct note: *What the fuck?*

Confused, I do both. I have a cup of tea and pretend nothing is out of the ordinary. I chat with Luke and Madison about everyday matters. For all appearances, I'm sitting in our family room. In reality, I'm skating on a pond covered in thin ice, fearing it'll crack and yank me to a cold murky bottom. I didn't want the opportunity to learn so much about breast cancer. I don't want to learn how strong I can be. I want to return to an ignorant state, in a land without radiation, catheters, encroachment, and pain. Most of all, I want the needles out of my body.

Logically their presence makes sense. The needles serve a purpose. They're part of the greater good. I should focus on that, rather than dwell on the trap that snared me. I must focus on the days ahead of me. I have to envision a future that doesn't include breast cancer. Worthwhile when spotlighted, nonetheless my repulsion runs deep, and must be shared and acknowledged. My situation is insufferable. I need confirmation. Inhabitations, those rules governed by correctness, seep from the punctures of my breast. I go to the bedroom to study the results of my treatment. I call for my daughter and husband to follow me.

Madison opens the bedroom door. She sees me half-naked. Her hand flies to her mouth.

"Oh my God," she screeches when she sees Niña Lola. "My poor mama."

Her arms immediately embrace, careful, fearful of the surgical steel protruding from my breast. She gives comfort and understanding and thirsting for kindness. I quaff it.

Luke wants to take a photograph. I refuse. This was not something I want to keep in an album. *And here's me getting ready for the barbeque.*

I receive a hefty dose of kindness from my family. I top it off with a full dose of pain medication. Only one catheter causes Niña Lola to writhe in pain but it does a good job of it. Without looking at a clock, I know when the four-hour lapse between dosages approaches.

We carry on with our typical schedule. Night falls. I look at the bed in confusion. I enjoy sleeping. I adore my thick pillow top mattress but presently it doesn't seem like an object I can rest upon.

"Would you like to sleep on the lazy boy?" Luke asks. The lazy boy is in the basement. "Zack and I will bring it in the bedroom."

"I should do okay in the bed."

"You move around a lot," he says with a grimace.

It's true. Morning finds me in a tangle of sheets. I often hunt for my pillow and my hair stands on end. We look at each other. I think we both imagine my breast impaled in the mattress. I can't envision myself falling asleep.

"The chair is awkward and heavy. don't bother. I won't sleep tonight." Luke looks horrified. I place my hand on his arm. "Don't worry, my mind won't allow me to hurt myself by tossing and turning."

We go to bed. I stare at the ceiling. I never sleep on my back. I can't understand how people can. It feels stiff and unnatural. Actually, I feel like a stiff. My hands fold over my stomach and, although my eyes close, images fire in my head. It was quite the day.

I don't remember surrendering to sleep, but I do. I wake up and everything is as it should be. The nibs are in place. Sleep didn't spear me into the mattress. I feel well rested. The surgery weakened my body. It made demands and overrode the trepidations of my mind.

My father always said: "You do what you have to."

His words made people sound strong and invincible. Daddy never fully explained the adage. You do what you have to because life takes away choices and leaves only one selection. You're no stronger than a cornered rat. Beneath the illusion of strength, lies weakness and fear. If you manage to get out of the corner and survive, fear and weakness slink from the room, leaving pride in their place.

*J*ARRIVE THE following morning to find only Mrs. Adams in the waiting room. It seems odd not to hear the chatter of a bevy of women. Mrs. Adams huddles into a corner with her daughter. They're talking quietly, their heads almost touching. The normalcy of the scene leaves me wondering if my feelings of pain and fear are histrionic.

How stupid is that? I question if she's made of a stronger material, a thicker fibre that allows her to withstand more. Should I try to do better? Should I peel my weakness and find courage? Am I making a big deal out of nothing?

Does it matter? Life is not a test of strength. Life is a series of experiences. Emotions are permissible. Sentiments make us human. Fear, repulsion and anything else I suffer is allowable. I chastise myself. It doesn't do any good. I want to be strong and unaffected. I can be such an idiot sometimes.

Luke and I take the seat across from them. Our proximity makes the room feel smaller. "How are you doing?" I ask.

"I'm holding up."

Sometimes you can't expect more than that.

Abby, her daughter says: "Mom showed me what they did to her. Oh my God."

Is that the classic response? Is that what Doctor Martin hears when he whips out his photographs for audiences to see. Does he enjoy doing it, because he thinks he's a god?

I can't imagine Mrs. Adams baring her breast for her daughter. Perhaps we aren't as different as I thought we were. Knowing they live in a village about forty-five minutes from the hospital, I ask: "Did you have any trouble getting in?"

"No. It was easy. We're staying at the lodge."

"Lodge, what lodge?"

"During brachytherapy you can stay at the lodge next door. They offer you a room with a bed, dresser and television set and a private bathroom. Didn't your nurse tell you about it?"

I find out that she did. I must have still been under the influence of drugs. Another Alzheimer moment. I wonder what else is lost to me. Time wise, it's only an hour. However, when you can't knit moments together, the size of the hole is astounding. What must it be like to live a life bombarded by holes? I think of my grandmother. She died of Alzheimer's. I saw it ravish her. I felt pity, but didn't truly understand her days until I had a hole of my own. And my hole is only little and explainable. Granny didn't have a little hole. She had an abyss where all her recent memories lay lost to her. How did she find the strength to open her eyes every morning? Her days must have been so confusing. I couldn't even pretend to be sure footed if bewilderment rocked my world.

Mrs. Adams is uncharacteristically chatty. I begin to warm up to her. I find out that she likes animals, especially horses. Her voice softens when she speaks of her grandchildren. She's trying to keep up with technology. She's succeeding. A small tablet rests on her knees. Enthusiasm and love surround her as she shows me images of cherished ones. When she speaks of her garden, her eyes sparkle. We both admit to subscribing to seed catalogues. Winter is long and barren. Dreams shorten the dreary months.

We're having an intense conversation about green garden products when they call my name.

My second treatment is the same as the first. My conversation about Easter continues with a brunette technician.

On the drive home, I laugh when Luke tells me Abby confided in him. "It seems her mother has been talking non-stop since having the procedure done. She's never quiet for a moment. Abby asked me if I had something for a headache. Her face lit up when I pulled out an Advil."

"I guess it's hard to deal with a chatty mother when you're used to a quiet one."

"Abby said her mother rarely takes drugs. She assumes the morphine is making her anxious."

"That and the needles piercing her chest. I personally like her on drugs. She's warmer and looser."

I don't admit I'm relieved the procedure affected her. I don't take joy in her unease. I only crave verification of my feelings. As I said before, I can be such an idiot sometimes. Why do feelings need corroboration? If one person feels emotions, are they less deserving and poignant than the emotions of many?

$\mathcal{M}$Y THIRD AND final treatment is taking place at three o'clock in the afternoon. I eat my lunch and watch the minutes tick by. I want the catheters out; I don't want them out. Do you know what I'm getting at? That's right, I'm a chicken ka-boob.

For the most part, I like being a human being. I can't imagine life as a dog, or worse yet a cockroach. However, there are times I despise our intimate relationship with time. We can't sever ourselves from the past. We often wallow over musty mistakes and long lost opportunities. The future can fill us with dread. We understand causality. Imagine the liberty if one faces a future unmindful of what will unfold. I finish my lunch. Drink my coffee. I walk upstairs and prepare to leave for the hospital. I brush my teeth and hear the music from *Jaws*. It amplifies what's about to take place. People tell me I'm lucky to be imaginative. I usually agree but, unfortunately, creativity amplifies moods. It's a great gift when you're cheerful and hopeful. I often hear Julie Andrews as Maria von Trapp sing Rodgers and Hammerstein's *The Hills Are Alive*:

> *The hills are alive with the sound of music*
> *With songs they have sung for a thousand years*
> *The hills fill my heart with the sound of music*
> *My heart wants to sing every song it hears*
>
> *My heart wants to beat like the wings of the birds*
> *that rise from the lake to the trees*
> *My heart wants to sigh like a chime that flies*
> *from a church on a breeze*
> *To laugh like a brook when it trips and falls over*
> *stones on its way*
> *To sing through the night like a lark who is learning to pray*

I go to the hills when my heart is lonely
I know I will hear what I've heard before
My heart will be blessed with the sound of music
And I'll sing once more

However, when frightened and apprehensive, imagination is an unnecessary accessory. I wish I could lock it up and retrieve it at a safer time. It comes in unexpected bursts. Mine is visual, with audio accompaniment. Negative situations bring bursts that fracture reality.

The music from *Jaws*.

The splattering of blood, dripping down white walls.

The yelp of a nurse as she holds the catheter up in the air with my breast still attached to it. "Never seen that happen before," she remarks as she flings my boob off the skewer. "They're a hundred and twenty-five dollars apiece," she explains, as she wipes the surgical steel clean.

The OOO of my mouth as it looks at the gaping hole in my chest. "I was never told this could happen!!!"

"Ready to go?" my husband asks.

"Ready," I squeak.

We arrive to hear the technician arguing on the phone with someone. It doesn't take long to decipher the one-sided conversation.

Doctor Martin isn't coming in to remove his handiwork. He's out of town and refuses to return to the hospital. The nurse doggedly tries to change his mind. Her voice starts angry, but turns resigning.

I pretend not to hear the conversation. When my treatment ends, the technician tells me to go next door. It's a small cramped room. Not the setting I imagined when I envisioned the removal of my gigantic needles. My trepidation has caused them to grow five sizes larger. They're now harpoons. Two nurses wait for me.

"Don't be afraid. It won't be as bad as you think it will be," one of them assures me as she smiles brightly. Her nametag reads Marthe. Her voice tells me she's the one who argued with the doctor.

The second nurse, Lisa, is younger. The green undertone to her complexion tells me she's inexperienced. I sit at the end of the examination table. The steal trolley holding alcohol and dressing squeaks as it rolls alongside of me. Marthe begins by removing the rubber nibs that hold the catheters in place. Her hair is freshly washed. I can smell her shampoo. Her watch ticks loudly. She's right handed. She wipes each puncture mark with alcohol. The stinging sensation causes my body to recoil from her.

"I'm a bleeder," I say, knowing that the next step is the removal of the five catheters. I feel they deserve a warning. I imagine the wall will look like a Jackson Pollock painting when she's done.

"You won't bleed," Marthe replies with absolute certainty.

Cleaning the area stings like hell. I'm afraid of embarrassing myself when she tugs the catheters out. I fear the scream will last a long time. I will myself to remain stationary and quiet. Pretend you're brave, I order myself.

Lisa takes hold of my hand and squeezes gently. Her hand is wet. "It's almost over," she says. There are times when almost doesn't count. Particularly the moment prior to nearly over.

A quick glance at the cart shows me my blood has already begun to flow. The white cotton baton Marthe used to clean me is red. I glance down at the skewers. They resemble the ones used for barbequing, especially when Marthe fits them into a steel casing. It's a relief. The casing attaches them to one another. One pull will pry them from my chest.

"Ready?" Marthe asks. Beads of sweat moisten her forehead.

I brace myself. "Ready."

Lisa, the green nurse, changes colour. She's now white. I fear she'll pass out. Maybe we'll enter unconsciousness together.

Marthe holds the skewers firmly. Her face looks determined. She pulls swiftly. The needles are out. Blood splatters, but it doesn't hurt. The intimidating music was unwarranted. My mind made the situation worse than it is.

It's over. Niña Lola looks blue and puffy. She has ten holes in her but she'll survive the experience. Breathe, Niña Lola, breathe.

After I'm dressed, I hurry to the waiting room where I see Mrs. Adams. "It's not as bad as you think it will be."

I guess I don't learn lessons well. I hope it goes as well for her as it did for me.

I never find out because I never see the woman again. After that day, our paths diverge. Oddly enough, months later, I'm in a restaurant in Manhattan. I hear my name. I turn around and see Abby. She asks how I'm doing. I say well. I ask about her mother. She too is doing well.

Suzanne sees me leave the change rooms. She smiles broadly and holds up a crown.

The crown is gaudy and cheap but its glued rhinestones catch the light and the effect is dazzling.

I'm sure it comes from the dollar store. How many little girls' hands touched it as they chose their tiara, as they dreamed of transforming into a fairy princess? This crown's destiny differs drastically from other coronets. It's not meant to be worn by little girls who envision faraway lands, filled with castles and princesses and princes. It doesn't represent a trip to a pretend land. Instead, it hails women who endured cancer treatment and who are returning to the real world.

"Come over here," Suzanne yells, her voice echoing in the empty room.

I walk over. She places the crown on my head.

"You look beautiful, my Queen," she exclaims.

It's my coronation. There are no women filling the waiting room to witness the event. There are no hands clapping in celebration. There are no yells of best wishes bouncing off the walls. The room is silent.

Mrs. Adams is being de-kaboobed. The new cancer patients are at another hospital.

I close my eyes. I see Connie, Francine, Darcy, Elizabeth. I see the faces of the women I passed in the hallway. I feel the presence of the women I met, cared for and admired. The walls embrace these women because heart-rending moments leave a lasting image. They're gone, but I see their smiles and hear their best wishes, for my heart embraced them and it will never let go.

Suzanne's arms encircle me. "Congratulations, it's finally over."

It's over. I leave the hospital. I now know why my assigned path didn't feel right. My body did submit to its fate. My skin is cut and burnt. My chest, branded. So many strangers handled me. I lost count of them. However, the blue dots never touched my soul, my heart, or my spirit. Those belong to me alone.

I think back on the pink zippy woman I encountered a lifetime ago. "I have another year," she whispered, in a tone implying she might not be as lucky next time around.

I am not that woman. I walk down the hallway. My feet are in perfect alignment with the blue dots. I will not lose my way.

"I have a lifetime," I roar to the empty halls. I hear a noise. I don't look back.

☙ Epilogue ❧

*D*ARCY IS SITTING at a table in a far corner, secluded from others. As I walk towards her, I see two coffee cups in front of her. One is a large double, double and the other is an extra large, triple, triple. I reach her, sit down, and grab the biggest cup.

I think of coffee as it spurts from her nose. I think of an egg as it runs down a man's finest suit. I think of lumpectomies, mastectomies, and hands, so many unfamiliar hands. Images bolt through my mind at lightning speed. I feel almost dizzy.

When we needed someone to understand our circumstances, we were there for each other.

Our circumstances have changed. Will we drift apart?

Of all the women I met, I like Darcy the most. She's tough, aggressive and can be difficult. But aren't those who challenge the very ones who make you feel alive and force you to think?

We shared so much but what we shared might rip us apart. When she sees me, does she think of breast cancer, of pain, of experiences best forgotten? Our journey is over. Will its conclusion mark the ending of our friendship?

My eyes become watery. I dare not blink. If I do, tears will course down my face. I suddenly blurt: "I hope we will always be friends."

I didn't plan to say the words aloud. I have the absurd habit of expressing myself in a voice only I can hear. Words are for sharing. Sometimes what should be shared remains silent and still. My thoughts barged out of my internal world. They embarrass me.

True to form, Darcy replies: "You're such an ass clown. I'm sitting across from you even though you must have the world's worst haircut. Of course we will always be friends."

I laugh. I do have the world's worst haircut but it doesn't matter because I'm sitting across from a dear friend. Cancer had the power to bring us together but it doesn't have the strength to rip us apart.

A friend is one to whom one may pour out all the contents of one's heart, chaff and grain together, knowing that the gentlest of hands will take and sift it, keep what is worth keeping and with a breath of kindness blow the rest away.

— ARABIAN PROVERB

Acknowledgements

Big thanks to my mother, husband, daughter and son, who are always there, even when "there" is not so nice. Special thanks to Connie Mc-Parland who saw something in *Hard Lumps* that she liked, and Michael Mirolla for editing my work. Appreciation to David Moratto who created what I sought but could not envision. I also want to thank my friends and family for being who they are. Last, but not least I want to thank the doctors, nurses and technicians who made an unbearable situation bearable.

About The Author

Nancy-Gail Burns, author of *Insidious and Jolted*, lives in Gloucester with her husband, daughter, son, two cats and a dog. She is currently at work on her next novel.

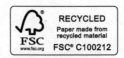

RECYCLED
Paper made from
recycled material
FSC
www.fsc.org   FSC® C100212

Printed in February 2014
by Gauvin Press,
Gatineau, Québec